The Good Pharmacist

What People Are Saying About "The Good Pharmacist"

"Every pharmacist and student pharmacist should read this book."

Cynthia L. Raehl, Pharm.D., Professor and Chair of Pharmacy Practice, Texas Tech University

"Finally, someone has studied the care side of pharmaceutical care. The Good Pharmacist gives us a 360 degree look at what it takes to be a pharmacist caregiver."

John A. Gans, Pharm.D., APhA Executive Vice-President & CEO Emeritus

"The Good Pharmacist provides confirmation and incentive to become even better in patient care. Put simply – it is a must read!"

Abby Caplan, Pharm.D., Clinical Coordinator, Kerr Health

"I highly recommend this book to any pharmacist who wants to be better."

Douglas E. Miller, Pharm.D., ASHP Leadership Award Recipient (2009)

"This book defines and gives insight into what a pharmacist should strive to be."

John Reinhold, Pharm.D., CGP, FASCP, Consultant Pharmacist

"I would want the pharmacist filling my prescription or my family's prescriptions to have read this book."

Linda A. Paterniti, RPh, Director of Pharmacy, Regional Cancer Center

*"Drs Kelly and Sogol have done the profession
a huge favor by discovering and writing about
what it takes to be a "good pharmacist."*

William E. Smith, Ph.D., Pharm.D., Professor of Pharmacy, Virginia
Commonwealth University

*"The book precisely details the factors necessary for any
pharmacist to improve their practice skills and interaction
with patients."*

Richard C. Messnick, JD, MHA, RPh, Pharmacy Manager, Pick 'N"
Save Pharmacy

*"The authors have given retail pharmacy a wonderful guideline for
hiring and employing pharmacists that was never there before."*

Brian Phillips, RPh, Target Pharmacy

*"This book provides understanding for patients, insight for
pharmacy students, and perspective for practicing pharmacists."*

Lisa A. Padgett, Pharm.D., Regional Clinical Manager, Kerr Health

*"The Good Pharmacist is a must read for
students and pharmacists alike."*

Steve M. Caddick, Pharm.D., Owner, Westchase Compounding
Pharmacy

The Good Pharmacist

Characteristics, Virtues, and Habits

William N. Kelly and Elliott M. Sogol

WILLIAM N. KELLY CONSULTING, INC.

OLDSMAR, FLORIDA

The Good Pharmacist: Characteristics, Virtues, and Habits
Copyright © 2011

International Standard Book Numbers
978-0-615-39321-6

Printed in the United States of America

Library of Congress Catalog-in-Publication Data
Kelly WN and Sogol EM
The Good Pharmacist – Characteristics, Virtues, and Habits. © 2011.
Includes bibliographic references and index.
Control Number 2010912593

To order go to: http:/www.thegoodpharmacist.com

William N. Kelly Consulting, Inc.
2147 Warwick Drive
Oldsmar, Florida 34677

Book Design by Brion Sausser: http:/www.bookcreatives.com

Dedication

This book is dedicated to the many "good pharmacists" who make patients the center of their daily practice.

Foreword

The Good Pharmacist is for those who care about the use and dispensing of medication, which is the primary professional responsibility of the pharmacist. The use of the term "good pharmacist" is common in pharmacy, but it has never been clearly defined. No matter how elusive, it is our collective aspiration to be considered a "good pharmacist."

Drs. Kelly and Sogol have provided us with a 360-degree view of this aspiration from the perspective of physicians, nurses, patients and other pharmacists. They have identified from their experiences the essential qualities of a "good pharmacist." The characteristics, virtues, and habits they have identified are central to the training, hiring and development of future "good pharmacists."

This book is based on a five year study beyond the clichés that "good pharmacists" are born, not made', and 'I know a "good pharmacist" when I see one.' The book should be essential reading for those of us who are pharmacists, leaders in the pharmaceutical profession, and educators of pharmacists. The authors' insights help us understand how others who use and need our services discover what makes a "good pharmacist." These are our customers and we need to listen to them.

The heart of the book is Chapter 2, "What Pharmacists, Doctors, Nurses and Patients Think." This chapter discusses the outcomes of the study and what each of the four groups say are the qualities of a "good pharmacist." Patients, for example, describe caring as an essential ingredient in building an effective therapeutic alliance. The authors challenge us to think about caring—the other half of pharmaceutical care—asking us whether this quality can and should be taught, measured, or made an admission criteria. Drs. Kelly and Sogol make the case for the centrality of caring in creating a successful therapeutic alliance that improves the patients' medication use and therapeutic outcome.

The book also focuses on two primary practice areas of pharmacy—community and hospital practice. In order to be a good communicator (a basic characteristic of the "good pharmacist"), a pharmacist should be directly accessible to the patient, which needs to become the standard especially in our community and hospital sites.

In Chapter 4, "good pharmacists" take the stand, defining in their own words what is considered essential in their practice. The words "fast and accurate" did not make their list. Critical words like "caring, teacher, problem solver" were more commonly used to describe their daily practice. The authors introduce us to visible patient-centered care, which the Institute of Medicine has made one of its six domains of quality.

The case is clearly made that if pharmaceutical care and medication therapy management become the standard of each pharmacist's practice, the quality of medication use will significantly improve. This will require the pharmacist to assume responsibility for their patients' therapeutic outcomes and to worry about how well their patients do. The book provides a tool for the assessment of a "good pharmacist", which allows practicing pharmacists to evaluate their strengths and weaknesses.

The authors outline steps for pharmacists to follow in using this tool to develop themselves into a "good pharmacist." It also asks readers to identify and nominate other "good pharmacists." They also discuss the necessary changes in the profession's environment that might facilitate developing visible patient-centered pharmacy practice as the standard in American pharmacy.

There are two major professional priorities: first, developing standards for measuring the quality of pharmaceutical care, and second, financial incentives to provide such quality pharmaceutical care. For only what is being evaluated and paid for gets done in our society.

This book challenges our thinking and moves us beyond our comfort zone. Medications have become the primary form of treatment today. We are currently developing personalized medication treatment plans. This coupled with new medications and biologics in the approval pipeline show great promise for the treatment and control of disease. In *The Good Pharmacist* the authors have identified the areas of pharmaceutical quality care that still need to be developed and standardized.

To date this book is the best effort to describe the "good pharmacist" and to identify characteristics to strive for as a new standard for pharmacist practice. This book is essential reading for student pharmacists, educators, and professional leaders who need to move the profession to a point where the "good pharmacist" is not an exception but the rule.

John A. Gans, Pharm.D.
Immediate Past Executive Vice-President
American Pharmacists Association

Preface

*Compliments like "What a good pharmacist!" raise that par-*ticular pharmacist above others that presumably are not as 'good', yet the qualities distinguishing a "good pharmacist" remain obscure. Indeed, sometimes when we ask what makes a pharmacist a "good pharmacist," the answer is as elusive as: "I don't know, but I know one when I see one."

Knowing the characteristics, virtues and habits of "good pharmacists" is important for several reasons. First, it is the key to providing proper education and training to student pharmacists. Second, knowing what makes a "good pharmacist" can help practicing pharmacists improve the care they deliver. Third, it can help managers and supervisors in their hiring decisions. And fourth, it can help move the profession closer to patient-centered care.

We performed a casual five-year study with the sole purpose of defining the elusive concept of the "good pharmacist." The results of the study are the basis for this book. In performing this research, we primarily asked questions such as: What is "good"? Who decides which pharmacists are good? And, who cares?

The latter question deserves further elaboration. At the time of the study, William Kelly was a full and tenured professor at the Mercer University School of Pharmacy that at the time enrolled 120 students a year, but had 1800 applicants. Based on grade point average (GPA) and scores in the Pharmacy College Admission Test (PCAT), 360 applicants made it to the next cut. The Assistant Dean for Admissions determined that all 360 students would likely be able do the academic work. That left three students to interview for every position available. After interviewing, the school accepted 120 students. Through questioning and observation, the faculty determined which applicants from the pool to accept into the school. Yet there were no written (or spoken) criteria by which to choose one applicant over the other. Shouldn't there be a better way to do this than an interviewer's whim? What if the qualities of a "good pharmacist" were the central focus of the criteria?

We know that pharmacy is a science and knowledge-based profession. Most schools of pharmacy expertly pass on academic knowledge to our pharmacy graduates. But pharmacy is more than that - its fundamental social purpose is to help patients.

An outcome-based curriculum would begin with what every graduate should know, and with the qualities the faculty desire in each graduate. Quite obviously, we should want each graduate to be a "good pharmacist!" Shouldn't applicant selection committees include the characteristics, virtues, and habits of a "good pharmacist?"

Elliott Sogol served on the admissions committee at the Campbell University School of Pharmacy and chaired the graduate program admissions committee. The numbers at this school were comparable. Also, this author helped develop a set of questions for the admissions committees of some schools of pharmacy that would be used in addition to GPA and PCAT scores. The interview questions and procedures emphasized an applicant's motivation, oral and written communication skills, problem solving, and caring. Applicant selection and curriculum committees should include the characteristics, virtues, and habits of a "good pharmacist." This book can help improve the selection process and the education and training of student pharmacists.

Furthermore, this book intends to:

- Help increase the visible patient-centered care delivered by pharmacists.

- Influence the upper management of pharmacists in institutional and community pharmacies.

- Help pharmacy supervisors understand the value of letting pharmacists practice visible patient-centered care.

- Identify some pharmacists named "good pharmacists."

- Identify those who named a "good pharmacist."

- Offer an opportunity to identify other "good pharmacists."

Therefore, the intended audience for this book includes pharmacy faculty, student pharmacists, practicing pharmacists, and managers and supervisors of pharmacists. Perhaps even patients will be interested in this book, as it can help and encourage them to expect more from their pharmacists and seek out those who deserve the elusive label of a "good pharmacist."

Acknowledgments

We would like to recognize and thank our mentors for the time and effort they spent to train our minds and model the behavior of true health care professionals and scholars. In particular we'd like to recognize the support of the late T. Donald Rucker, Ph.D., a productive scholar and friend, who advised us on the book and recommended our collaboration. We would also like to thank our families for their support. Dr. Sogol would like to specifically thank Lori, Whitney, Sydney and his parents for their continued encouragement.

We would also like to thank our peer reviewers, whose comments have helped edit the book: John A. Gans, Charles D. Hepler, Douglas E. Miller, Cynthia L. Raehl, N. Lee Rucker, William E. Smith, and William A. Zellmer.

About the Authors

William N. Kelly, Pharm.D., FISPE has over forty years of experience in various health care settings including: acute care, ambulatory care, long-term care, home health care, academia, and the government. He is president of William N. Kelly Consulting, Inc., a company devoted to advancing medication safety and the practice of pharmacy, and Vice-President of Scientific Affairs with Visante, a pharmacy consulting company in Minneapolis, Minnesota.

Before starting his company in 2005, Dr. Kelly was the Chair of Pharmacy Practice and a tenured professor at the Southern School of Pharmacy at Mercer University and Guest Researcher at the Immunization Safety Branch of the Centers for Disease Control and Prevention (CDC). Prior to those appointments, he was Assistant Vice-President and Director of Pharmacy at Hamot Medical Center, a 550-bed acute care health-system and clinics in Erie, PA.

He earned a BS in pharmacy from Ferris State University, a doctor of pharmacy (Pharm.D.) and a residency certificate in clinical pharmacy from the University of Michigan. Dr. Kelly also completed a fellowship in executive management at the Leonard Davis Institute of Health Economics at the University of Pennsylvania. He also completed graduate work in pharmacoepidemiology and biostatistics at McGill and Emory Universities, and is a fellow of the International Society for Pharmacoepidemiology (ISPE).

Dr. Kelly has published over 85 peer-reviewed manuscripts, ten chapters in books, and has presented his work nationally and internationally. He is the author of *"Pharmacy: What It Is and How It Works"* (CRC Press, 2002, 2007, 2011), and *"Prescribed Medications and the Public Health: Laying the Foundation for Risk Reduction"* (Haworth Press, 2007). He is the past chair and member of the United States Pharmacopeia's (USP's) Expert Committee on Safe Medication Use, and a past member of the National Coordinating Council on Medication Errors and Prevention.

Elliott M. Sogol, Ph.D., RPh, FAPhA is the Group Manager – Professional Services for Target, overseeing clinical pharmacy services, education, and professional development programs for Target pharmacists and pharmacy technicians. In addition, Dr. Sogol functions as Target's liaison for schools of pharmacy and pharmacy associations. He is an adjunct faculty member at the University of Florida, the University of Minnesota, the University of North Carolina, and Campbell University.

Besides his role at Target, Dr. Sogol is the Science Officer for the American Pharmacists Association (APhA). In this role he collaborates with others on issues about science policy, legislation affecting pharmacy and healthcare, and the growth of the profession through applying science into practice. He is also a researcher and trainer for the APhA Pathway Evaluation Program, a career planning program for student pharmacists.

Dr. Sogol spent 14 years in the pharmaceutical industry, most recently serving as the Director of Strategic Operations for the regional medical scientist (RMS) group in the US medical affairs division at Glaxo Smith Kline. Dr. Sogol also was the Director of Health Care Coalitions, and Director of External Professional Education

Programs. In addition, he was a faculty member at the University of Illinois and Campbell University Schools of Pharmacy for six years.

In 2003, Dr. Sogol became a Fellow in the APhA. He has also been honored with the Linwood F. Tice - Friend of APhA - Academy of Student Pharmacists Award. Other honors include the University of Wisconsin Graduate Excellence in Teaching Award and the Rennennbahm Teaching Award for Excellence at the University of Wisconsin - School of Pharmacy.

Dr. Sogol has served on the board of visitors for the University of Wisconsin - School of Pharmacy and the Dean's Advisory Board at the Chicago College of Pharmacy – Midwestern University. He is a past board member of the National Council on Patient Information and Education. He was the chairperson of the Board of Directors of the North Carolina Museum of Life and Science and state wide chairperson of the North Carolina Math and Science Education Network. In addition, Dr. Sogol has presented his work nationally and internationally.

Dr. Sogol earned a BS in pharmacy, MS, and Ph.D. in pharmacy with a minor in business from the University of Wisconsin - School of Pharmacy in Madison.

Contents

Chapter One

Who is a "Good Pharmacist?"

*Compliments like "What a good pharmacist!" raise that par-*ticular pharmacist above others that presumably are not as 'good', yet the qualities distinguishing a "good pharmacist" remain obscure. Indeed, sometimes when we ask what makes that pharmacist a "good pharmacist," the answer is as elusive as: "I don't know, but I know one when I see one." Few would argue with that. For example, if you met pharmacists Stephen Dendiak, Louis Mundy, or Bob Brashear, you would no doubt say they are "good pharmacists." Let's meet them.

Stephen Dendiak (Atlanta, GA)[1] – "He was good at what he did. That's why he was my pharmacist," said Stephen's physician. A patient said: "He had a personal touch." Another said: "He was compassionate and caring." And yet another patient said: "He always gave people extra service. He would tell you about drug interactions and problems you could expect. You never felt rushed dealing with Stephen. If I asked a question he couldn't answer, he would get the information and call me back." Stephen's characteristics, virtues, and habits look like this:

Characteristics: *knowledgeable*

Virtues: *caring, compassionate, patient, just, kind*

Habits: *responsive*

Note: A characteristic is a distinguishing trait, feature, or qual-ity that is not a virtue or a habit. A virtue is a specific moral quality regarded as good or meritorious. A habit is a something done often and easily.

Louis Mundy (Tyrone, GA)[2] - Also known as "doc" by his patients, Louis often returns to his pharmacy after-hours to help patients. "He does it for many people much of the time," says a loyal patient. People like Louis because they know him and he knows them. "He answers the phone and hears my voice and knows it is me," says another patient. People like Louis's pharmacy because "you are treated like a human being – not a number." Mundy also has provided prescriptions to some patients on credit, which "has been a blessing to many folks around here."

Characteristics: *knowledgeable*

Virtues: *caring, friendly*

Habits: *available*

Bob Brashear (Iverness, FL)[3] – Bob knows the names of all of his patients. "Everyone is a friend here," says Bob. "It means a lot to look someone in the eye and show them compassion." Such attention and personal contact draws legions of loyal customers. One patient says: "Bob is never too busy to talk to you and answer questions. In bigger pharmacies, you pay your money, get your pills, and walk out with no personal instructions."

Characteristics: *knowledgeable*

Virtues: *caring, friendly*

Habits: *available*

Characteristics, Virtues, and Habits – "Good pharmacists" have common characteristics, virtues, and habits. Summarizing those of Steven, Louis, and Bob, we arrive at a list that looks like this:

Characteristics: *knowledgeable, sincere*

Virtues: *caring, compassionate, patient, just, kind, friendly*

Habits: *responsive, available, dependable*

Although these qualities sound reasonable and might be the essence of a "good pharmacist" per se, the sample is too small (n of 3) to draw any conclusions. Therefore, identifying what makes a "good pharmacist" needs more work. The following chapters explore who decides and what makes a "good pharmacist." In addition, we've included a self-assessment evaluation to see if you might be a "good pharmacist." (see Chapter 7).

But first, let's explore a key question

Who Cares What It Takes to Be a Good Pharmacist? The first group who cares is the hardworking faculty at over 125 schools and colleges of pharmacy. Pharmacy faculty would be wise to design an outcome-based curriculum focused on the characteristics that make a "good pharmacist," and the academic knowledge it takes to graduate.

Although pharmacy is a science and knowledge driven profession, "caring" deserves more than lip service in the curriculum. It truly needs to be taught as well. A compelling question for pharmacy schools is: Are you concentrating too much on the science and clinical knowledge of the curriculum, and not enough on the attributes and components of caring that are left to adjunct preceptors and postgraduate mentors?

Another, equally important question is: Where do these preceptors receive information on and training in caring if they did not receive it in school? At a minimum, we recommend that faculty assess their curricula (didactic and experiential) against what we have discovered about "good pharmacists." How well are the school's adjunct preceptors modeling what it takes to be a "good pharmacist?" How do you know for sure? How are the preceptors evaluated? Is it important the preceptor makes sure that all the check marks are completed on the didactic experiential side or should this be more?

Preceptors know that they have an important role to help mentor and show by example how to be a "good pharmacist," and therefore they are the second group who cares what it takes to be exactly that. A "good pharmacist" who is a preceptor has the professional responsibility to not only teach, but also advise, critique and provide opportunities to learn in a safe environment.

Practicing pharmacists are the third group with an interest in knowing what it takes to be a "good pharmacist" so they can improve their practice to advance patient care. Taking the evaluation in chapter 7 will help a pharmacist discover where her or his strengths lie with regards to the elusive label of being a "good pharmacist."

Finally, we think those who supervise and manage pharmacists should know the qualities of a "good pharmacist" so they can help pharmacists grow professionally and receive satisfactory recognition. For the same reasons, we feel it is important for those in upper management of local, state, and national chain pharmacies (who often are not pharmacists) to know what they should strive for in hiring and retaining pharmacists in their employment. Owners of independent pharmacies and pharmacy directors in health systems also should review the information to discover if they and their staff are moving toward being a "good pharmacist."

A "good pharmacist" has a greater potential for performing a patient-centered practice environment that provides for increasing patient adherence, communication between patients – prescribers – pharmacists, and the opportunity to help patients make informed decisions about the medications they take, and about OTC products, food, nutrition, health, and wellness.

A good pharmacist helps the patient (or caregiver) to know:

1 How to use the medication, especially how to use administration devices like metered dose inhalers. The patient should be able to demonstrate correct use in the pharmacy.
2 What drugs/foods to avoid, e.g., antacids, grapefruit juice, etc, when taking medication.
3 How to recognize whether the medicine is working as planned (e.g., symptom resolution within three days from UTI antibiotic) or to know that there should not be any change in how the patient feels (e.g., statins)
4 How to recognize serious and common adverse events, side effects, etc.
5 What to do (whom to call) about non-appearance of therapeutic effect or appearance of adverse effect
6 Essential follow-up such as returning for monitoring tests.

–Doug Hepler[4]

If you wish to recruit the patient as an active participant in her or his own care, it is not enough to hand the patient a medication information leaflet. A "good pharmacist" should take a yellow highlighter pen and mark the information that is essential for their patient's success in taking the medication. A "good pharmacist" would also begin follow up (a phone call) consistently, at least with high risk patients.[4]

The Institute of Medicine (IOM) reports have the facts on record

– the quality of health care in the United States is not acceptable. There are problems with access, quality, and cost, and medication use is a leading problem. Pharmacists should be constantly vigilant for ways to prevent harm and promote rational drug therapy. We need "good pharmacists" so, at the end of the day, these pharmacists have optimized their contributions to helping patients make the best use of their medication while facing the least risk.

Summary – Some pharmacists have distinguishing qualities that make them "good pharmacists." Discovering these distinguishing qualities can help in teaching student pharmacists, improve the care pharmacists provide, and help patients make the best use of their medication.

Chapter Notes

1   "Stephen Dendiak 59, Caring Pharmacist." The Atlanta Journal-Constitution. Obituaries. September 12, 2004.
2   Lewis, S. "Just a House Call Away. Not Guided by Clock, Tyrone Pharmacist Always Ready to Help Customers, Friends." The Atlanta Journal-Constitution. Living Section – M-1. September 23, 2001.
3   "Everyone Is a Friend at This Pharmacy." St. Petersburg Times. Section 2D. November 13, 2006.
4   Personal Correspondence between William Kelly and Charles Hepler. July 13, 2010.

Chapter Two

What Pharmacists, Physicians, Nurses, and Patients Think

Pharmacists have a history of reaching out to other healthcare professionals and patients to develop a baseline of understanding about our roles and responsibilities to our profession. Often these surveys are in response to political and professional practice issues, or are undertaken by a third party looking into the profession.[1-5] This chapter discusses the objectives, methods, and results from our study on what four important groups think are the qualities of a "good pharmacist."

Study Question – What do pharmacists, physicians, nurses and patients consider the characteristics, virtues, and habits of "good pharmacists?"

Objective – Our cross-sectional, multi-stakeholder, descriptive survey was designed to reach out to groups that interact with pharmacists regularly to discover the qualities (characteristics, virtues, and habits) of a "good pharmacist." Our rationale was that the different groups interacting regularly with pharmacists are seeking characteristics that promote a professional and visible patient-centered interaction.

Hypothesis – The hypothesis was that the different groups would mention different qualities of the "good pharmacist" depending on the specific needs of the respective group. The primary goal was to discover if there are qualities that run across and between groups that interact with pharmacists, or if pharmacists are viewed differently by these groups.

Each participant was asked to list three adjectives (in single words), in order of importance, that describe a "good pharmacist." These were categorized based on a pharmacist the participant said was a "good pharmacist." Our survey was independent of the work environment where the pharmacist was employed, as respondents could name a "good pharmacist" from a community, institutional or other practice setting.

Methods – To explore this topic, we used a qualitative research design that provided information and data to address the research question. Early decisions were made to reach a sample of participants in a cost effective and efficient manner. Taking this into consideration, a convenience sample was used for the first phase of this research. Participants were selected based on accessibility to the authors and convenience of delivery of the survey.

Limitations of a convenience sample are well known. For example, the information uncovered may be biased based on the sample chosen. However, to address this limitation, we delivered the survey through several vehicles. The survey was sent via email, provided at local pharmacies, through interviews at national meetings, through web-based survey access, and through contacts within professional organizations.

The first phase of the project was a means to gather qualitative data to provide a hypothesis for future research. This convenience sample is the basis for the results provided in this book.

Qualitative inquiry – strategically, philosophically, and therefore, methodologically – aims to minimize the imposition of predetermined responses…so people can respond in their own words.

–Michael Quinn Patton[6]

Survey Completion – Paper surveys (see sample in the back of the book) were either faxed or mailed to the authors, while the on-line version provided an electronic submission process. All survey data was analyzed by grouping responses based on similar interpretation of responses to the open-ended questions.

Table 2.1 below provides the number of participants in each of the four groups that completed surveys. Tabulation included 111 usable responses.

Table 2.1
Number of Participants by Discipline

Database – The database (MS Access) listed the most common themes that emerged from each of the four groups taking part in the survey. Of interest are the more than 100 adjectives used to describe a "good pharmacist."

Table 2.2 below summarizes the number of different adjectives listed by participant group.

Table 2.2
Number of Different Adjectives Identified by Discipline

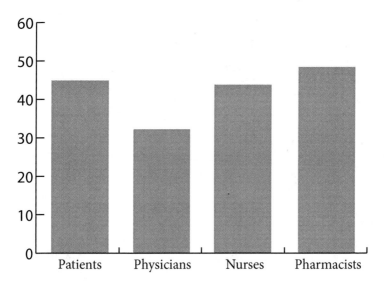

Analysis - Qualitative analysis techniques were used to group similar adjectives and statements to reveal the key qualities of those considered "good pharmacists." The analysis included a search for definition of terminology to verify likeness of words and the difference in interpretation of the adjectives provided. Working with a rhetorician, respondent results were categorized into major domains.

Results - In general, results provide data across five domains of a "good pharmacist." These domains were created to provide parallelism across the responses. Each domain listed below provides the rationale and descriptor of the domain with the adjectives that were categorized into each domain.

There is overlap of the adjectives listed in the first two categories, as many could fit under multiple domain headings. However, we grouped these based on our interpretation of added written information provided by respondents on open-ended comments. These qualities are not listed in any specific order.

General Qualities of a "Good Pharmacist"

A "GOOD PHARMACIST" IS AN EXPERT:

Respondents understand a "good pharmacist" to be someone who possesses expertise – someone with comprehensive and authoritative knowledge and skill (up-to-date, logical, smart, analytical, explanatory, expert, a teacher, clinically competent, intelligent, respected, evidence-based, knowledgeable, and current).

A "GOOD PHARMACIST" IS A PROFESSIONAL:

Respondents understand a "good pharmacist" to be someone who exudes professionalism (team-oriented, leader, informative, well-spoken, collaborative, organized, professional integrity, and a good communicator).

A "GOOD PHARMACIST" HAS A SOLID WORK ETHIC:

"Good pharmacists" are perceived to be people who present a strong work ethic – they intrinsically believe hard work is virtuous and "good" (careful, prompt, diligent, detail oriented, informed, fast, accurate, meticulous, focused, efficient, hard working, resourceful, precise, results-oriented, attentive, discerning, dedicated, thorough, precise, hard-working, focused, aware, problem-solver, effective, timely, and initiative).

A "GOOD PHARMACIST" HAS STRONG MORAL CHARACTER:

Pharmacists are perceived to be of a higher moral make-up than the average population (mature, supportive, accessible, sense of humor, thoughtful, gregarious, warm, affable, pleasant, tenacious, joyful, nice, honest, dependable, judicious, personable, patient, responsible, considerate, conscientious, trustworthy, sincere, observant, inclusive, incorruptible, visionary, cautious, enthusiastic, good tempered, kind, friendly, and sincere).

A "GOOD PHARMACIST" IS PATIENT ORIENTED:

Pharmacists see beyond the prescription to the individual (polite, accessible, interactive, faithful, neighborhood-centric, contributing, straight forward, respectful, compassionate, approachable, non-judgmental, empathetic, listens, involved, visible patient-centered, concerned, helpful, understanding, courteous, responsive, and available).

Specific Qualities of a "Good Pharmacist"

Table 2.3 on the following page lists the adjectives in rank order of frequency by participant group. Note that each respondent group included two groups of adjectives as positive characteristics: one being knowledgeable, and the other being empathy, caring, or compassionate.

Table 2.3 Specific Qualities of a "Good Pharmacist" Listed by Respondent Groups

Pharmacists (n=36)	1. EMPATHY, CARING, OR COMPASSIONATE
	2. KNOWLEDGEABLE
	3. GOOD COMMUNICATOR
	4. DEDICATED
	5. PATIENT
Physicians (n=21)	1. KNOWLEDGEABLE
	2. GOOD COMMUNICATOR
	3. EMPATHY, CARING OR COMPASSIONATE
	4. CONSCIENTIOUS
	5. THOROUGH
Nurses (n=27)	1. KNOWLEDGEABLE
	2. EMPATHY, CARING OR COMPASSIONATE
	3 FRIENDLY, ATTENTIVE
	5. PRECISE OR ACCURATE
Patients (n=27)	1. KNOWLEDGEABLE
	2. EMPATHY, CARING OR COMPASSIONATE
	3. ATTENTIVE
	4. PRECISE OR ACCURATE
	5. FRIENDLY
All (n=111)	1. KNOWLEDGEABLE
	2. EMPATHY, CARING, OR COMPASSIONATE
	3. FRIENDLY
	4. PRECISE OR ACCURATE
	5. CLINICALLY COMPETENT
	6. GOOD COMMUNICATOR
	7. ATTENTIVE

The information presented provides insight into the thoughts of some pharmacists, physicians, patients, and nurses about the qualities embodied by a "good pharmacist." The adjective "knowledgeable" was a dominant characteristic chosen by all four groups. All four survey groups also selected empathy, caring and compassionate (grouped) as key virtues. These qualities focus on a visible patient-centered process where the pharmacist has the necessary knowledge while also showing genuine care for patients' health and well being.

This suggests that just having the knowledge of the profession and learning the skills of empathy are not the only qualities that pharmacists or others consider when thinking about the "good pharmacist." Taking responsibility to work with patients is needed to help make informed decisions on medications that affect the health and well being of patients and the community.

Summary – The pharmacists, physicians, nurses, and patients we surveyed mentioned the following as the general qualities of the "good pharmacist": being an expert, professional, having a strong work ethic, strong moral character, and being patient oriented.

Chapter Notes

1   Robers, PA. "Job Satisfaction Among US Pharmacists." Am J Hosp Pharm. 1983, 40: 391-399.

2   Knapp, DA; Knapp, DE; Evanson RV. "Determining the Role of the Community Pharmacist." Am J Pharm Educ. 1965; 29: 274.

3   Barnett, CW and Kimberlin, CL. "Job and Career Satisfaction of Florida Pharmacists." Fla Pharm J. 1986; 50 (April): 8-10.

4   Desselle, SP and Tipton, DJ. "Factors Contributing to the Satisfaction and Performance Ability of Community Pharmacists: a Path Model Analysis." J Soc Admin Pharm. 2001; 18: 15-23.

5   Mott, DA; Doucette, WR; Gaither, CA; Pedersen, CA; Schommer, JC. "Pharmacists' Attitudes Toward Worklife: Results From a National Survey of Pharmacists." J Am Pharm Assoc. 2004; 44: 326-336.

6   Patton, MQ. Qualitative Research & Evaluation Methods. Thousand Oaks: Sage Publications., 2002.

Chapter Three

Key Qualities That Make Pharmacists "Good"

Like physicians and nurses, pharmacists are at the moral center of healthcare.[1] Pharmacists should be in a unique covenant with patients. What would you say is the difference between the relationship of a flight attendant and a passenger versus the relationship of a pharmacist and a patient? The major differences are: the pharmacist-patient relationship is personal, professional, and discreet, and should result in a lasting bond as compared to a period in time provided while on an airplane where the relationship ends when one disembarks from the airplane.

> *The covenant between the patient and the pharmacist goes like this: If you (the pharmacist) help me make the best use of my medication and remain discreet, I (the patient) will give you my respect, trust, and cooperation.*
> *–William N. Kelly*

What Patients Want from Pharmacists – Besides wanting their prescription filled correctly, patients want respect, recognition, and a sense of significance, but most of all they want their pharmacist to be available, friendly, and caring. Caring is an essential element of being a "good pharmacist," and is "one of the preconditions for building an effective therapeutic alliance with patients."[2]

What is Goodness? – Goodness is a virtue that is the best part, essence, or valuable element of something. Goodness involves having a heart, mind, and character for helping others. It is the companion of the virtue kindness.

Kindness puts others at ease and shrinks from giving discomfort. Being kind may include not complying with the letter of the law if it concerns a grave patient need. For example, although dispensing a prescription without proper renewal from a prescriber is technically illegal, providing a few doses until she or he can be contacted in the morning would be an act of kindness by the pharmacist. Note: This assumes the pharmacist has queried the patient to determine if the medication is still needed, effective, and safe.

> *No act of kindness, no matter how small, is ever wasted.*
> *–Unknown*

Based on our survey and interviews, we hypothesize the key qualities of a "good pharmacist" are: being knowledgeable, caring, friendly, precise and accurate, clinically competent, a good communicator, and attentive.

Knowledgeable – Having superb knowledge of pharmacy, pharmaceuticals and biologics, disease states, and applying this knowledge to patient care was a unanimous characteristic among all four survey groups (pharmacists, physicians, nurses, and patients). Pharmacists should not just use her or his knowledge to dispense a medication properly. Also important is: 1) making discoveries about the patient and her or his disease, health status, and medication-related problems; and 2) teaching the patient about the medication so each individual patient can make an informed decision about her or his therapy. Simply dispensing medication without performing these value-added services relegates a pharmacist to the category of "super pharmacy technician."

> *Knowledge itself is power.*
> –*Sir Francis Bacon, English Author, 1561-1626*

When pharmacists use their knowledge in all three domains (dispensing, discovery, and counseling), they are more than likely taking responsibility for the patient. The difference between a "good pharmacist" and other pharmacists is the way they see their role. The "good pharmacist" respects patients and sees her or his role as helping patients make the best use of their medication, while other pharmacists see their role as dispensing medication without much need to interact with patients.

However, when patients speak of the "good pharmacist," they are not talking about the pharmacist's knowledge and technical expertise. They are thinking about the virtues of caring and friendliness, the characteristic of good communication, and the habit of being attentive.

Caring – Caring is a surrogate for the essential ethical virtue beneficence. It is the characteristic most patients want in a pharmacist: personal caring and a genuine relationship. Caring shows interest and is a generosity of spirit and the enemy of selfishness. Caring involves being available and connecting with patients, forming a true bond, helping, and having patience. When you show patients you care, they become transformed. Co-suffering by feeling the patient's vulnerability and acting on it is evidence of compassion. A true bond forms when the pharmacist goes through the experience with the patient.

Empathy is a practical competence.
–Peter Drucker, Author (1909-2005)

"Good pharmacists" care. Sadly, many pharmacists are preoccupied with processing prescriptions and medication orders quickly. The question we should pose is whether and how the profession could and should motivate pharmacists to be caring? Should this be an integral part of the scope of practice? What does the profession think about these questions?

While there is a need to include measurements that look at the "number of prescriptions" per hour, day, week, or year, we should also measure the delivery of patient care. If pharmacists were reviewed and rewarded for achieving a specific patient based outcome (a disease state or loyalty based on the care provided), an outcome that supports practicing as a "good pharmacist," this alone could drive the profession in the right direction.

Friendliness – Besides knowing their patients and acting in their best interest, "good pharmacists" feel empathy and understanding towards patients, and patients respond. This does not always happen in every patient encounter, but the "good pharmacist" is always friendly, even if the patient is not. After all, not feeling well often affects a patient's behavior (see Chapter 5). Personalized pharmacy service is the best we can deliver – a genuine affect in the patient-pharmacist relationship. This will happen readily when the pharmacist is friendly.

According to our survey results, patients want a closer relationship with their pharmacist. However, to be a patient's friend, a pharmacist must be available, and not stuck or hidden behind the pharmacy counter, computer, or in the hospital or health-system pharmacy.

Hence being approachable, patient, and never condescending becomes rather important. If the pharmacist approves the dispensed medication, but bypasses positive interaction with the patient, she or he is not fulfilling her or his obligation to the patient. The patient then owes the pharmacist nothing more than her or his fee, because the pharmacist does not view the patient as a friend, but as the impersonal recipient of a unit of production. The pharmacist who is patient-centered and friendly has a better chance to easily extract important clinical information relevant to the patient's medication regimen.

Precision and Accuracy – Precision and accuracy are a given within the profession, and clearly something every pharmacist strives for, whether in measuring, dispensing, or establishing a patient's dose. This also applies to communicating drug information to other health professionals and to patients. Despite our best efforts, medication errors continue, seemingly unabated. All pharmacists should be pushing for a change from a culture of blame to a culture of safety, and for more tools that will help prevent medication errors.

In pharmacy, being "close" is rarely good enough.

Clinically Competent – Three of four survey groups selected clinical competence as a requirement for a "good pharmacist". Of course, not all pharmacists practice clinically. Many pharmacists are still stuck (many by choice) in the preparation and dispensing modes, and many do not interact face-to-face with patients, physicians, and nurses.

Clinical Competence is the capability to perform acceptably those duties directly *about* patient care.
                                    –Webster

Until a tipping point is reached when most pharmacists practice clinically, interact with patients directly, and receive an incentive for doing so, those outside the profession will view the pharmacist simply as the dispenser of medication.

A Good Communicator – The physicians and pharmacists we surveyed listed good communication as an important skill of the "good pharmacist." Clear and concise communication with patients about their medication can help avoid serious problems.

Not understanding the medication, not knowing how to take the medication properly, not knowing how to use a device, and not knowing potential dangers, can lead to serious patient problems. But communication is a two-way street – "good pharmacists" listen to their patient's concerns and identify medication-related problems (MPRs). Also, "good pharmacists" take the next step and communicate with other health care professionals to make sure all are informed of the situation.

Pharmaceutical care involves one patient, one pharmacist at a time.[3]
                                    –Cynthia Raehl

Being a good communicator means you must be available to patients. In the community pharmacy setting, the best pharmacist-patient communication is when the pharmacist accepts the prescription, interviews and counsels the patient about his or her medication, and identifies MRPs as an integral part of processing the prescription. Although the pharmacist will need to check the dispensing for correctness, qualified pharmacy technicians (preferably certified) can do everything else. Technicians are given responsibility for the "filling" of the overall prescription process. This recommended procedure increases the time the pharmacist spends with the patient, and solidifies patient satisfaction and loyalty.

In hospitals and health-systems, the goal should be that most patients say "yes" when asked if they interacted with a pharmacist during their stay. It is even better if the patient remembers the pharmacist's name. However, many patients do not even know there are pharmacists in hospitals and health-systems.[4]

"A reasonable goal (in the hospital or health-system) would be to have a pharmacist meet every patient receiving substantial medication therapy."[5] When doing this, the "good pharmacist" would identify herself or himself as a pharmacist, give the patient a personal business card, and leave behind helpful, easily understood printed information about the medication discussed.[6]

"Good pharmacists" (see Chapter 4) tell us they are teachers. They teach patients about their medication and they teach student pharmacists, pharmacy interns, and pharmacy residents how to be a "good pharmacist." A good teacher speaks in terms their audience understands, from patients who need word pictures, to complex examples in teaching future practitioners, and always checking for understanding.

Attentive – In our survey, nurses and patients placed being attentive high on their list of habits that make a pharmacist "good." According to Webster, attentive means paying attention, being observant, considerate, respectful, devoted, thoughtful. Its companion virtue is faithful. "Good pharmacists" are faithful by being available, reliable, and attentive to their patient's needs.

One area where pharmacists can improve being attentive to patients is over-the-counter (OTC) medication counseling. Patients often wander up and down the OTC aisle looking over various OTC medications, scratching their heads, and wondering what they should buy for a problem they or a loved one is experiencing. This often takes place close to where the pharmacist is standing behind the counter with his or her head buried in the computer. A "good pharmacist" would be attentive, and immediately go out and help the patient purchase the appropriate OTC remedy. The discussion should include non-therapeutic options or advisement for the patient to see a physician, should the situation warrant. Should this be a scope or standard of practice issue?

> *Those who are silent, self-effacing and attentive become the recipients of confidence*
>
> *– Thornton Wilder, American Writer (1897-1975)*

Summary – The pharmacists, physicians, nurses, and patients we surveyed told us that "good pharmacists" are knowledgeable, caring, friendly, precise and accurate, clinically competent, good communicators, and attentive to their patient's needs. There should be nothing more important to a pharmacist than a patient, be they someone who the pharmacist has cared for over the years or a first time patient.

Chapter Notes

1 Pellegrino, ED and Thomasma, DC. The Virtues in Medical Practice. Chapter 3 – Medicine as a Moral Community. Oxford University Press. New York, 1993.

2 Berger BA. "Building an Effective Therapeutic Alliance: Competence, Trustworthiness, and Caring." Am J Health-Syst Pharm. 1993; 50: 2399-2403.

3 Raehl CA. "One Patient, One Pharmacist." Am J Hosp Pharm. 1994; 51: 1928-1930.

4 Chrymko, MC, and Kelly, WN. "Are There Really Pharmacists in Health-Systems?" Am J Hosp Pharm.1989; 46: 2000–2001

5 Zellmer, WA. Let's Talk. The Conscience of a Pharmacist. American Society of Health-System Pharmacists. Bethesda, MD, 2002. Pages 101-102.

6 Zellmer, WA. Improving the Image of Pharmacists. The Conscience of a Pharmacist. American Society of Health-System Pharmacists. Bethesda, MD, 2002. Pages 97-106.

Chapter Four

What "Good Pharmacists" Tell Us

Further insight into what makes a "good pharmacist" was provided by the nomination portion of the survey forms that allowed people to name professionals they considered to be "good pharmacists," and to provide an example of when and how the pharmacist they named displayed the qualities making her or him a "good pharmacist." After review of these examples, we interviewed eleven pharmacists over the telephone, asking them what they felt made them a "good pharmacist?" Here is what they said:

Gerald Briggs – Huntington Beach, CA. BS Pharm., Washington State University (1968). Mentor: William Smith, Ph.D., Pharm.D.

"My success as a pharmacist is based on the word "s.p.i.r.i.t." The S stands for specialized. Selecting a clearly defined practice area allowed me to become an expert.

The P stands for problems, presentations, and publications. Identifying medication-related problems in patients is an opportunity for pharmacists to show what they can do. Presentations give me credibility within my work site, while publications give me credibility outside my work site. The first I stands for involvement. I am involved directly in the care of patients. I help with patient concerns. The R stands for research. The research question comes from clinical practice and thus is practical. The second I stands for carrying out solutions to the patient problems identified. The T stands for teaching students how to be good clinical practitioners."

Characteristics: *knowledgeable, teacher*

Virtues: *helpful*

Habits: *problem-solving*

Brad Cooper – Erie, PA. Pharm.D.. Purdue University (1984). Mentor: Judy Jacobi, Pharm.D.

"I learned early from my mentors that they took an interest in their patients. They put forth extra effort and thought a lot about their patients, not only during the day, but sometimes even after hours at home. I develop rapport with physicians and nurses and take care of many issues they bring to my attention. I want patients to receive the best care possible."

Characteristics: *sincere*

Virtues: *faithful, just*

Habits: *responsible*

Cecily DiPiro – Charleston, SC. Pharm.D. University of Georgia (1995). Mentor: Rusty May, Pharm.D.

"I care a lot about my patients. I put their needs first. I follow through and do what I have promised. Providing good patient care is important to me. Patients can rely on me. I make sure patients have what they need and I problem solve for them. I spend the necessary time with my patients and love teaching them. I win their confidence. Each day I come into work and leave work with a smile."

Characteristics: *teacher*

Virtues: *caring, faithful, joyful*

Habits: *problem solving*

Eli (Elisha) Guadalupe – Nashville, TN. BS Pharm. Samford University (1993). Mentor: David Ferrell Gregory, Pharm.D.

"I put myself in the shoes of the patient. I respect them and treat them the way I would like to be treated. I take time to answer questions, and if I do not know the answer right away, I always get back to them when I say I will, or talk to someone who can. No job in pharmacy is beneath me – I even have done deliveries. I do whatever it takes to help the patient."

Characteristics: *teacher*

Virtues: *respect, patience, faithful*

Habits: *persistence*

Richard Manny – Tampa, FL. Pharm.D.. University of Texas (1984). Mentor: Sid Pridgen, BS Pharm.

"I am a teacher and patient advocate. I hold a patient's hands and listen. I always make myself available and take time with patients. I believe in patients and in the profession. I teach pharmacy students to observe patients for clues that reveal needs or medication-related problems. I want students to see the "whole patient." I am joyful when helping to resolve a patient's problem."

Characteristics: *teacher*

Virtues: *kind, faithful*

Habits: *listening, problem-solving*

Ray Marcrom – Manchester, TN. Pharm.D.. University of Tennessee (1972). Mentor: H.D. Marcrom, RPh

"Patients matter to me, regardless of income, social status, or race. Patients always deserve my best and I want to be their friend. I also try to go the extra mile for patients, like calling a physician when someone else would not take the time to do that. I am willing to come into the store early if a patient cannot get there later. I also think it is important to take the role of a servant and to buy into and accept that idea. I want to make a difference in patients' lives. There is much art in pharmacy – not just science."

Characteristics: *servant*

Virtues: *respect, caring, friendly*

Habits: *responsible*

Melissa Somma McGivney – Pittsburgh, PA. Pharm.D.. University of Pittsburgh (1998). Mentor: Joseph Bechtel, RPh

"Patients are my priority. Listening to patients is critical to being a good practitioner and an important skill for pharmacists. I try to identify a patient's needs, even if the need has nothing to do with medication. Sometimes you need to help connect patients to other providers that can help. I also try to have rapport with physicians, nurses and other pharmacists."

Characteristics: *connector*

Virtues: *respect, caring*

Habits: *responsible, listening, problem-solving*

Tenny Moss – Florence, SC. BS Pharm. Medical University of S. Carolina (1972). Mentor: Herman Cox, BS Pharm

"My primary purpose is to be a good teacher. So I spend time making sure patients know about their medication. We counsel every patient. Providing counseling to patients involves teaching. I feel we have a responsibility to be faithful to our patients. I always try to do my job well. It's also important to teach pharmacy students how to care and problem solve for patients. I also teach physicians about how to write prescriptions customized for patients and they appreciate that."

Characteristics: *teacher, knowledgeable*

Virtues: *faithful, patience*

Habits: *responsible, problem-solving*

Sheila Neiman – Brooklyn, NY. BS Pharm. Long Island University (1980). Mentor: Richard Blum, MD

"I have high awareness of a culture of safety that should exist to protect patients. It started when I was working in community practice and has carried over to my health-system practice. I also love patient contact. I have always felt that I can make a difference in their care. Some patients fall between the cracks and need extra time and attention. My workplace is the last resort in New York City, and we try to give what every patient needs in care and hope."

Characteristics: *advocate*

Virtues: *justice, caring, respect*

Habits: *responsible*

Francis Unrein – Plainville, KS. BS Pharm. University of Kansas (1951). Mentor: Charlie Harkness, RPh

"I took care of all the local people who needed medication and provided advice about their medication. I explained to patients why they were on the medication as their physician usually did not take the time to do that. Patients relied on me and trusted me. I was a friend, available, and attentive to their needs. I delivered prescriptions to the elderly who could not get out. I am still known to many as "doc."

Characteristics: *teacher*

Virtues: *caring, faithful, friendly*

Habits: *service*

April Vanis – Atlanta, GA. BS Pharm., University of Georgia (1997). Mentor: Mary Anne Hawkins, Pharm.D..

"Patients come first. I am dedicated and like to help patients. I am motivated by making a difference in people's lives. I always try to give extra care and attention. I want people to feel better, so I try to give each person time. Genuine caring is critical to what we do as pharmacists."

Characteristics: *dedicated, servant*

Virtues: *helpful, caring, patience*

Habits: *attentive*

From this field study, we learned that "good pharmacists" are not thinking of efficiency and skill when asked what makes them a "good pharmacist." Rather, they are thinking of the empathy, kindness, and the graciousness that she or he brings to all her or his patients.

Table 4.1 on the following page summarizes the top characteristics, virtues, and habits "good pharmacists" tell us they are using.

Table 4.1 Qualities Mentioned by Some "Good Pharmacists"

No.	Qualities	No. of Times Mentioned
1	CARING	6
1	FAITHFUL	6
1	TEACHER	6
4	RESPONSIBLE	5
5	PROBLEM SOLVER	4
6	RESPECTFUL	3
6	PATIENCE	3
8	KNOWLEDGEABLE	2
8	LISTENER	2
8	HELPFUL	2
8	SERVANT	2

Table (4.2) summarizes the list of qualities nominators felt good pharmacists have (see Chapter 2).

Table 4.2 Qualities Mentioned by Nominators

No.	Qualities	No. of Times Mentioned
1	KNOWLEDGEABLE	54
2	EMPATHY, CARING, OR COMPASSION	35
3	FRIENDLY	14
4	PRECISE OR ACCURATE	13
5	CLINICALLY COMPETENT	12
6	GOOD COMMUNICATOR	10
6	ATTENTIVE	10
8	CONSCIENTIOUS	7
9	HELPFUL	5
10	KIND	5

When comparing and contrasting the two tables, we see good pharmacists telling us they are doing more than being knowledgeable, caring, friendly, precise and accurate, clinically competent, a good communicator, and attentive. They are also taking responsibility for patients and are problem solvers and good teachers (of patients and students). It is understandable that knowledge and good communication are down on their list, something they take for granted.

Summary – Good pharmacists tell us they are: caring, faithful, teachers, responsible, and problem solvers. In short, they are clinically competent and provide visible patient-centered care and concern.

Chapter Five

Visible Patient-Centered Care

The field study has shown that providing visible patient-cen-
tered care is a desired characteristic of a "good pharmacist"

What is Visible Patient-Centered Care?

The Institute of Healthcare Improvement (IHI) says that patient-centered care is "care that is truly patient-centered, considers patients' cultural traditions, their personal preferences and values, their family situations, and their lifestyles. It makes the patient and their loved ones an integral part of the care team who collaborate with health care professionals in making clinical decisions."

Patient-centered care puts responsibility for important aspects of self-care and monitoring in patients' hands — along with the tools and support they need to carry out that responsibility.

Patient-centered care ensures that transitions between providers, departments, and health care settings are respectful, coordinated, and efficient. When care is patient-centered, unneeded and unwanted services can be reduced."[1]

This is a long and tedious definition. Here is a much simpler one: *patient-centered care* makes the patient the central focus, places emphasis on patient participation, considers the patient's perspective, and tailors care to the patient's needs and preferences. It should be visible and measurable.

Visible patient-centered care focuses on the patient – not on how care is delivered. For example, it is much too common today for a health care provider to meet with a patient without saying her or his name, their title, or even why she or he is there. Some "would have us believe that completing the task alone is enough. Quality is measured by how skillfully and efficiently the task is performed. But from the patient's perspective, every task is more than the delivery of medical services."[2]

> *One of the essential qualities of the clinician is interest in humanity, for the secret to the care of the patient is in caring for the patient.*
> *–Francis Weld Peabody, MD*[3]

The Institute of Medicine (IOM) made patient-centered care one of six domains of quality. According to the IOM, "research shows that orienting the health system around the preferences and needs of patients has the potential to improve patients' satisfaction with care as well as their clinical outcomes."[4]

The Patient – Being a patient can be scary. Patients' fears may originate from a bad health care experience, but usually stems from lack of medical knowledge, a high-level of reverence for health professionals, and being timid.

Confusion and bewilderment occur when health professionals use unfamiliar medical terms. Because patients sometimes do not understand, they feel they must place their trust in the professionals who care for them.

Most health care professionals do not recognize the wide communication gap between professionals and patients. Most health care professionals will never be able to understand and recognize what patients endure with illnesses and the health care system unless they themselves become a patient.[5] Many patients do not take their medication. Some tolerate serious side effects because they do not connect the problem to their medication. Some patients do not even know the names of their medications. Some do not know why they are taking the medication, perhaps because their physician is busy preparing to see the next patient, or their pharmacist is too busy filling other prescriptions, or has a low priority for medication counseling.

Patient Needs – Pharmacists and student pharmacists need to understand patients rather than take them for granted. In the movie "The Physician," William Hurt plays a cardiovascular surgeon who says to his surgical residents – "Patients feel frightened, embarrassed, vulnerable, and sick, and most of all they want to feel better. Because of this, they place their faith in us. I can explain that until I am blue in the face, but you will never get it until you experience it for yourself."[6]

An injured lion still wants to roar
–Randy Pausch[7]

Medical care is far from being "user-friendly." Patients become frightened when they can't understand what health care providers are saying – the information is too technical or provided too rapidly. Terms used in discussion may be common to the health care professional, but unfamiliar to the average person. An example is that many hospitals and health-systems have signs that say "Radiology Department" while patients often look for the "X-Ray Department."

Patients can become embarrassed when asked to undress, made to wear revealing gowns, and discuss confidential matters. Some feel vulnerable because they know so little about health care. It is like a language they do not understand. Because of the education needed to be a health care professional, most patients are in awe of those who care for them. This lack of understanding has patients presenting their bodies, minds, and sometimes their dignity with an "I surrender" attitude. Some patients readily acquiesce – here I am, do whatever it is you are going to do to me – without questioning their medical treatment.

Patients have names – they are not the cabdriver with the gastric ulcer or the talkative women with hypertension. They come from different cultural backgrounds and have differing attitudes about being sick, seeking treatment, and their own role in implementing treatment regimens.

Patients can be passive, compliant, demanding, challenging, questioning, or cooperative. Most of all, they are sick, worried, and in need of our help.

Even patients who feel well have concerns about what medication (prescription and OTC) they are taking and why – especially if no one takes the time to provide the information they seek and provide a visible patient-centered safe environment.

Most patients want to demystify health care, have more control over their own destiny, and be identified as a person, rather than as another problem. They want their health care professionals to connect with them, understand their illness and their feelings; they want their health care professionals to care about them, not treat them like a number, and do their best at getting them well. Patients need and want understanding, reassurance, education, and choices.

> *There are five dimensions of care that every patient has*
> *the right to require of their encounters with the health*
> *care system. Don't kill me (no needless death). Do help*
> *me and don't hurt me (no needless pain). Don't make*
> *me feel helpless. Don't keep me waiting. And, don't waste*
> *resources, mine or anyone else's.*
>
> –Donald Berwick, MD[8]

Healthcare in the United States seems more concerned about the "what" and "why" of care, while patients prefer the "how" and "by whom." For example, the excessive waiting times many patients endure are unacceptable, but some healthcare providers do not recognize the importance of time and practice management to good patient care. Providing care is more about them than about the patient.

Evolving Pharmacy Practice and Its Relationship to Patient Care

Pharmacy practice in the United States has evolved through several practice models. Allow us to provide a quick historical account.

Compounding – The first apothecaries in the United States prepared medicine by incorporating the substances from nature into a tincture, syrup, tea, cream, ointment, suppository, or capsule. Pharmacists practiced artful pharmacy by making accurate, elegant, custom designed pharmaceutical products.

> *In the 1920s, 80% of the prescriptions filled in American*
> *pharmacies required knowledge of compounding.[9]*

Drug Dispensing and Drug Use Control – As large scale manufacturing of medicines by pharmaceutical companies grew, the art of pharmacy compounding dwindled. By the early 1960s, pharmaceutical companies produced most drug products prescribed by physicians. Thus, pharmacy practice emphasis shifted from drug preparation to drug dispensing. The simultaneous growth of third-party reimbursement for prescriptions added paperwork that impinged on pharmacists' time with patients.

> *Since any attempt to analyze the pharmacist's function must account for the patient's safety as well as his medication, one can reach a conclusion that the mainstream of pharmaceutical service is drug use control.*
> *–Donald C. Brodie, Ph.D.*[10]

Clinical Pharmacy – Pharmacy schools and some pharmacists became more clinically oriented during the 1960s by getting out of their hospital pharmacies and up on patient floors. This practice eventually became known as clinical pharmacy.[11] Clinical pharmacists advised prescribers in making drug therapy decisions and some achieved recognition as "drug experts" or "specialists." Between 1960 and 1980, a growing number of pharmacists with a doctor of pharmacy education (Pharm.D. degree) and completion of a pharmacy residency, practiced clinical pharmacy, mostly in hospitals and health care-systems (like HMOs).

Some roles of these early clinical pharmacists were to: be available for consultation with the physician when the drug was prescribed; recommend drug selection, the dose, and duration of therapy; and monitor the drug administration and effects of the drug. Physicians and nurses started to understand the benefits (to them and to patients) of having a clinical pharmacist available on the patient care unit. However, the customers of clinical pharmacists were rarely patients.

> *I also think of the clinical pharmacist as a pharmaco-therapeutic specialist. The important considerations, I believe, are his knowledge of therapeutics and the actions of drugs in humans.*
> –Donald E. Francke, DSc[12]

Pharmaceutical Care – In 1989, Hepler and Strand argued that clinical pharmacy represents a transition in pharmacists seeking self-actualization and their potential as professionals.[13] They appealed to pharmacists to accept preventing drug-morbidity and mortality as a primary responsibility. They also cautioned that applying clinical knowledge and skill (then known as clinical pharmacy) was not enough for pharmaceutical services. There needed to be a philosophy of practice and organization. This philosophy became pharmaceutical care.

> *If pharmaceutical care can prevent treatment failure or other drug-related morbidity or mortality, it is much more valuable than the services incident to selling a drug product.*
> –Charles D. Hepler, Ph.D. and Linda M. Strand, Ph.D.[14]

Consensus emerged on the mission of the pharmacist – to provide pharmaceutical care. Pharmaceutical care was defined as "the direct responsible provision of medication-related care for the purpose of achieving definite outcomes that improve a patient's quality of life."[15]

Caring, a long-standing virtue among nurses and physicians,

has been an understated part in pharmacy practice and education. Thus, caring is the dominant feature of pharmaceutical care. However, since introducing pharmaceutical care over twenty years ago, many pharmacists are still practicing without much face-to-face patient contact. For some, this represents a lost opportunity to show patients that pharmacists care and have more to offer than just the medication. For others, such as those practicing in mail-order settings, clinical pharmacy and pharmaceutical care is difficult to practice, given that there is no face-to-face patient interaction. This is not to say that pharmacists practicing in mail-order pharmacies are not concerned about patients, they just have limited opportunities to interact with patients.

The Patient-Pharmacist Relationship

At the center of discovering the qualities of a "good pharmacist" is the patient-pharmacist relationship. First, there must be a relationship, and second, that relationship must involve caring and trust.

Trust – According to Gallup polls before 1999, the public consistently rated pharmacists the most trusted professional.[16] In 1999, the survey added nurses who topped pharmacists for honesty and ethical standards. In 2009, the most trusted professional by the public was the nurse, but only one percentage point separated them from pharmacists.[17]

Understanding why the public rates pharmacists so high is elusive. Some say this is because patients do not get to know pharmacists well, while others say the high rating is because we do not charge for our advice. The truth is – no one knows. The profession would be wise to explore what the public thinks of us and why they trust us.

Patient Expectations – The public's high rating of pharmacists may be because of a low expectation of what pharmacists can provide beyond dispensing medications. Most patients have little knowledge of the pharmacist's extensive education and training. Our guess is that most patients feel the pharmacist's only role is to provide the medication. Many first-year student pharmacists have this same notion. Patients often judge pharmacists by accessibility, appearance, and communication skills. If the pharmacist hides behind the prescription counter, none of these expectations are met.

A community pharmacy study asked patients what they expected from their pharmacist.[18] The result was disappointing. Most patients did not even have an answer. After providing the patients with a list of possibilities, the top patient expectations of pharmacists were to: 1) fill the prescription correctly, 2) uphold confidentiality, 3) check for correct dosage, 4) check for drug interactions, and 5) check for drug allergies. Ninety-four percent of patients responded that it was important or very important that pharmacists showed they cared about them. However, only 40% of the patients and 50% of the pharmacists queried felt they had a close relationship with each other.

The 2008 *Pharmacy Satisfaction Digest Survey* of 71,000 households in 48 states discovered that patient trust resides in a personal relationship with the pharmacist.[19] The degree of trust varied by type of pharmacy with independent pharmacists scoring the highest. However, the range of "least trust" for all settings was 26-67%. We have a ways to go to increase patient trust.

Complaints About Pharmacists – From our surveys designed to uncover the qualities of the "good pharmacist," as a by-product of our research we also discovered some complaints about pharmacists. Several potential survey patients said they could not tell who behind the prescription counter was a pharmacist and who was a technician or a clerk – they all look about the same. One potential survey patient said, "I never get to talk with a pharmacist," while another said "I have never had a conversation with a pharmacist, so I'm afraid I cannot help." Another stated, "I have little contact with a pharmacist – they always seem too busy doing what they do behind the counter."

Another person said: "We can't properly answer the survey as we use mail order for our medications. Before that, a technician would ask us if we had questions. When I asked about a side effect, the technician went and asked the pharmacist then came back and gave me an answer." A recent survey revealed that only 36% of patients using a community pharmacy could name the pharmacist who filled their prescription.[20]

How can the profession do a better job of distinguishing who in the pharmacy is a pharmacist? Many pharmacists have exchanged their social identification (white coats and ties) to be more casual. Is this good?

Several nurses completing the survey expressed concern that pharmacists should be more available and approachable to help them. There are also concerns among state boards of pharmacy that pharmacists are not personally offering to counsel patients about their medication despite a legal requirement to do so.[21]

Fears of Patient Counseling

Patient counseling and pharmaceutical care are pivotal parts of pharmacy today. But we're reluctant to do it, we just weren't taught that way.

Talking with patients about their medications wasn't taught in schools of old. "It's the physician's job and not our own." That's what all of us were told.

And so we practiced for decades. Afraid of what we say might be used against us in legal proceedings some day.

But things have changed, responsibilities doubled. It is what we don't say today that gets us into legal trouble.

We're afraid to make our patients wait. We're afraid they may implore, "Twenty minutes for twenty pills, I'm going to another store."

Waiting and seeing the physician can take an hour or two. But for this most trusted health professional, complaints are relatively few.

The difference is the way patients perceive the value of the care they receive. If we provide counseling and pharmaceutical care, then complaints about waiting, they wouldn't dare.

But pharmacists are still reluctant to counsel as well as we could. We are afraid to assume the responsibilities that we all know we should.

And so we make up excuses like we don't have time to spare. If only we had more courage, we could practice pharmaceutical care.

–Richard A. Jackson, Ph.D.
Previously unpublished

The Pharmacist and Visible Patient-Centered Care

So what does it take to be a "good pharmacist?" Based on our survey results and from interviews with pharmacists named as "good pharmacists," it takes more than knowledge – a "good pharmacist" is all about the patient.

Caring – Good pharmacy practice involves a genuine interest in humanity. If true, do you as a pharmacist, student pharmacist, or pre-pharmacy student love and care about patients? Why? The answer to this question is a barometer for how you will perform your duties as a pharmacist.

Caring about patients is sometimes difficult for student pharmacists to grasp. The following exercise one pharmacy professor uses to enlighten his students can illustrate:

> The class is asked to close their eyes and think about the person they love the most — a husband, wife, girlfriend, boyfriend, mother, father, sister, brother, daughter, son, grandmother, grandfather, or grandchild. After a minute, the professor says, "Open your eyes and listen. Every time you interact with a patient – across the counter, or when they are in a hospital or health-system bed – pretend that patient is the person you love the most." The professor then asks, "If you do this, what will happen?" Students answered: "I would do my best." "I would make extra effort." "I would make sure they understood everything."

Accepting Responsibility for the Patient - "Good pharmacists" accept responsibility for their patients. They listen to and treat patients as if they were the most important person in their life.

The professor who devised the exercise to illustrate caring mentioned above, also makes responsibility part of his teaching. "How do you accept responsibility for the patient?" he asks. "How can you tell if the pharmacist is accepting responsibility for the patient?" The classroom became deadly silent. None of the 120 students raised a hand. The professor repeated the question and waited. Finally, one brave student said, "I think accepting responsibility for patients has something to do with worrying." Intrigued, the professor asked the student to explain her answer.

"Well," the student said, "if a pharmacist works all day, goes home and never worries about a patient, then that pharmacist probably is not accepting responsibility for her or his patients." This is exactly right — without worry, little responsibility is taking place.

Continued follow-up is another way for the pharmacist to accept responsibility for the patient. This includes discovering how well the medication is working and if the patient is experiencing any problems.

Helping Patients Make the Best Use of Their Medication – Our study of the "good pharmacist" also reveals that "good pharmacists" are interested in helping patients make the best use of their medication. This involves listening and goes beyond just answering questions and trying to identify, resolve, prevent or refer medication-related problems (MRPs). For further information on what it means to help patients make the best use of their medication, return to Chapter 1 and read the last part of that chapter.

The Patient's Story – Every patient has a story. The patient's story will reveal the MRPs. However, to gain clues about the MRPs, the pharmacist must win the patient's trust and listen. Trust begins in establishing a patient–pharmacist relationship. Trust evolves from kindness, friendliness, caring, empathy, honesty, justice, and confidentiality, and is strengthened by actions of past caring — all virtues of a "good pharmacist." A pharmacist, like any good listener, must listen with the whole mind and heart, trying to feel empathy for the patient's vulnerability. Probing questions should follow.

Summary – "Good pharmacists" are knowledgeable and care about their patients. They give patients their time and dispense sympathy and understanding along with the medication. The personal bond between the pharmacist and the patient forms the greatest satisfaction in pharmacy practice. "Good pharmacists" provide visible patient-centered care.

Chapter Notes

1   Patient-centered Care – General. Institute for Healthcare Improvement. http://www.ihi.org/IHI/Topics/PatientCenteredCare/PatientCenteredCareGeneral/. Accessed 1/8/10.

2   Frampton, SB; Charmel PA. Putting Patient's First: Best Practices in Patient-Centered Care. Jossey-Bass Publishers. San Francisco, 2008.

3   Peabody, FW. "The Care of the Patient." *JAMA*. 1927;88:877-882.

4   Patient-centered care. The Commonwealth Fund. http://www.commonwealthfund.org/Topics/Visablypatient-centered-Care.aspx. Accessed 2/3/10.

5   Rosenbaum, EE. A Taste of My Own Medicine: When the Physician is the Patient. Random House. New York, 1988.

6   Caswell, R. The Physician. Touchstone Pictures (1991). Based on citation #4.

7   Pausch, R. *The Last Lecture*. Chapter 1. Hyperion. New York, 2008.

8   Berwick, DM. "My Right Knee." *Ann Intern Med.* 2005;142:121-125.

9   Cowen, DL and Helfand ,WH. *Pharmacy*. Harry N. Abrams, Inc. Publishers. New York. 1990.

10 Brodie, DC. "Drug-Use Control – Keystone to Pharmaceutical Service." *Drug Intell Clin Pharm.* 1967;1:63-65.

11 Francke, DE. "Evolvement of Clinical Pharmacy." in: Francke, DE and Whitney,HAK Jr. eds. *Perspectives in Clinical Pharmacy; A Textbook for the Clinically-Oriented Pharmacist Wherever He May Practice.* Drug Intelligence Publications, Hamilton, IL, 1972:26–36.

12 Francke, DE. "Levels of Pharmacy Practice." *Drug Intell Clin Pharm.* 1976;10:534.

13 Hepler, CD; and Strand, LM. "Opportunities and Responsibilities in Pharmaceutical Care." *Am. J. Pharm Ed.* 1989; 53 (winter suppl.): 7S–15S.

14 Hepler, CD, and Strand, LM. "Opportunities and Responsibilities in Pharmaceutical Care." *Am J Hosp Pharm.* 1990;47:533–543.

15 American Society of Health System Pharmacists. Statement on Pharmaceutical Care. http://www.ashp.org/DocLibrary/BestPractices/OrgStPharmCare.aspx. Accessed 2/8/10.

16 Anonymous. "Ten In a Row." *America's Pharm.* 1999; 121 (Jan): 9.

17 Gallup Poll Votes Nurses Most Trusted Profession. December, 2009. http://www.medicalnewstoday.com/articles/173627.php. Accessed 2/8/10.

18 Smith, LL; Kramer, SV; and Kelly, WN. "Are Pharmacists and Patients Expectations of Each Other the Same?" *Georgia Pharmacy J.* 2004; Oct:20-22.

19 2008 Pharmacy Satisfaction Digest. Boeringer Ingelheim Pharmaceuticals. Inc.

20 Anonymous. "Pharmacy's Proximity Ranks as First, Survey Finds." *Pharmacy Times.* 2008; June: 2.

21 The Role of Patient Counseling in Preventing Medication Errors. NC State Board of Pharmacy. http://www.ncbop.org/about/Student%20Projects/PatientCounselingPreventingErrors.pdf. Accessed 2/8/10.

Chapter Six

Making "Good Pharmacists"

As stated earlier, we hypothesize from our study that "good
pharmacists" are knowledgeable, caring, precise and accurate, attentive, friendly, good communicators, teachers, and they take responsibility for patients. While we can look to the qualities listed by physicians, nurses, patients, and pharmacists, we need to ask a pressing
question. How do you become a "good pharmacist?" Are "good
pharmacists" born, raised that way, or can we influence this through
the admission, education, and training process? Are there turning
points where one begins to see the qualities and characteristics in
practice? Do mentors play a role in developing a "good pharmacist?"

Education

Let's start by examining how one undertakes the process to
become a pharmacist: from the preprofessional curricula, to the
application process, to the professional curricula, to graduation, to
licensure, and the steps (or leaps) between.

The preprofessional college curricula are often considered a
process that lays the foundation for the professional curricula.[1] Most
schools of pharmacy use student performance in the preprofessional
college curriculum as the basis for their ranking of applicants. It is
not known if or how the preprofessional college curriculum contrib-
utes to the making of a "good pharmacist." Perhaps one could look

at the courses in the humanities and social sciences as listed in the Accreditation Council for Pharmacy Education (ACPE) guidelines for preprofessional college curricula as a foundation for some of the characteristics and qualities of a "good pharmacist."[2] In addition, providing opportunities for leadership through local, state, national, and international, professional association student chapters, professional fraternities and sororities, and extracurricular activities.

A study by the American Foundation for Pharmaceutical Education (AFPE) provides a glimpse into why some students who have received educational grants and scholarships chose our profession. Many (57%) of the respondents said that mentors in high-school or early college courses played a key role in their thinking to continue their chosen career path in pharmacy.[3] Some respondents to the AFPE survey described a comment by a teacher or professor about their abilities that influenced their decisions. Early influences begin to help build a foundation of caring and passion for the profession that may then help to begin the basis of the qualities discussed earlier.

Admission Criteria and Selection

Does a school of pharmacy's admissions and selection process provide a link for an applicant to become a "good pharmacist?" The data collected in our survey seems to suggest that the admissions process, which so far mostly looks to didactic evaluation, should give equal value to criteria that address visible patient-centered care.

Each school of pharmacy has criteria on what makes a successful student in their program. Analysis of grade point average (GPA), standardized test data from the Pharmacy College Admissions Test

(PCAT), science and math abilities dominate the requirements for admissions. Intellectual capabilities, motivation, and decision making are criteria that are newer to the process used by admissions committees to identify who should be successful in the program.

The application process for admission to a school of pharmacy can be viewed as an entry into the profession – the first step in professionalizing a future pharmacist. Therefore, it makes sense that the criteria and admissions process should involve multiple layers of analysis. What type of process is asked of the applicant? Is this strictly a form to be completed, a check mark in the correct box? Does this represent what we are seeking in future pharmacists, or are we only looking at who can pay the tuition, master the academic curriculum, and graduate?

Taking all of this information into consideration, one could ask - Do schools of pharmacy look at characteristics that reflect the qualities of the "good pharmacist" found in our study? What types of graduates does the admissions committee envision? And last, but not least, do the current criteria guiding the selection process lead to admitting students who will become "good pharmacists?"

Are there questions in the interview process that address an applicant's inclination toward qualities such as precision and accuracy, caring for others, good communication skills, and attentiveness, friendliness, as well as a thorough, conscientious, and dedicated work ethic? Do these qualities need to be addressed, and if so, how should they be incorporated into the professional curriculum? It is not a matter of just stating them. It is vital to ask - can these qualities be seen in the preceptors that provide the experiential education? Discussions of where in the curriculum this can be included are important.

Submerged below the surface like an iceberg is the question whether virtue can be taught and whether the characteristics of the "good pharmacist" peek through the pre-pharmacy candidate even before she or he is admitted to pharmacy school.

The question though is how much weight is given to these areas. Is it more important that an applicant have the highest GPA possible with communication abilities that are modest at best, or that an applicant have a reasonable GPA (reasonable enough that the admissions committee has selected them to be interviewed) with excellent communication skills, a caring personality, showing motivation to help patients make informed decisions?

If we have a candidate pool to choose from, should we not weigh what we need in the profession from both the didactic and behavioral sides of the equation? If the chosen applicants display the beginning qualities of a "good pharmacist," and are then presented with the most appropriate educational courses, all – students, faculty, state boards of pharmacy, professional associations, and most importantly patients – will win.

In a recent presentation before the Multiple Owners Conference of the National Community Pharmacy Association (NCPA) in St. Thomas, VI, the Director of Human Resources for the Ritz-Carlton Hotel chain presented how his company provides service to its guests. He said the question people most often ask is "How do you train those employees of yours to be so pleasant and respectful?" His response is: "We do not train them at all to be that way. We only hire employees who already are pleasant and respectful."

The Disney Corporation provides superb service to its guests and is well known for training employees of other companies through Disney University. During our study, we inquired how Disney employees provide such superb service to their guests. We were told that, like Ritz Carlton, Disney screens potential employees to assure they have all the characteristics, virtues, and habits they need to be an employee before they hire them.[4] Disney basically uses two sets of screening questions. The first are "getting to know you questions" like:

- What customer service do you expect when you go out?
- What is the most important aspect of customer service?
- Do you enjoy being around children?
- Provide an example of teamwork
- Provide an example of a problem and how you solved it

The other questions are "what if" questions like:

- What would you do to welcome guests and spread some magic?
- What would you do if a child was afraid to go on a ride?
- What would you do if a child was too small to ride one of our attractions like Space Mountain?

The conclusion seems inescapable. It is much easier (and probably much better) to admit students to pharmacy school who already possess most qualities the "good pharmacist" needs rather than try to teach these characteristics, virtues and habits. Shouldn't applicants receive preference if they can provide some evidence of helping and caring work, volunteer work in health services, etc., in addition to good grades? Shouldn't there be something in the early curriculum to discourage students who do not care about helping people, i.e. the pharmacy equivalent of fecal exams and bedpan emptying for pre-med students?

DIDACTIC PROFESSIONAL CURRICULUM

The pharmacy current curriculum has been developed and established to ensure that future pharmacists have the knowledge to become medication experts. The curriculum not only looks to the profession's current needs, but also anticipates the critical knowledge base that will be needed to support the profession as it moves forward toward more clinical based, patient-centered care.

Of interest is that the curriculum changes over time to address the needs of the profession, patients, and the community. This swing, at times, may push too far or not far enough toward a specific topic or discipline within the profession. Some have proposed the curricula of the future will center around three roles: visible patient-centered care, population-based care, and systems management.[5]

How does instruction in medication therapy management (MTM) and other clinical care services help a student pharmacist become a "good pharmacist?"

In general, teaching how to complete the core element stages of MTM does not mean one cares for their patient. Rather, it is how the pharmacist integrates visible patient-centered care into the MTM process that determines if she or he is headed toward becoming a "good pharmacist."

As an example, a pharmacist can go through the motions of the core elements in working with an individual patient, document all the necessary interventions and complete a medication action plan with little or no caring – just "going through the process." In comparison, a pharmacist can go through the motions of the core elements, while at the same time providing explanations of the process, asking questions and listening to the patient's needs and concerns. The latter would most definitely would tailor the information to suit the individual patient and provide a medication action plan that will be implemented based on the care provided and the attentive nature of the pharmacist.

EXPERIENTIAL CURRICULUM

Applying the didactic knowledge of the profession to the practice environment is a critical art of the process that provides student pharmacists the opportunity to practice their skills and watch experienced practitioners. Experiential curricula have expanded to include competencies such as OTC counseling, explanation of inhalation devices, counseling on specialty pharmaceuticals, pharmacist administered immunizations (where allowed) and others.

While completing these competencies is important, a question arises if we are addressing how the competencies are achieved. In other words, are pharmacist preceptors providing the environment to become "good pharmacists" and displaying the characteristics and qualities that have been mentioned? No doubt many "good pharmacists" are also preceptors who provide guidance, mentorship, and trying to lead by example.

CURRICULAR OUTCOMES

For some student pharmacists, the primary curricular outcome is "passing the exam." For others it is the scientific inquiry and decision process - trying to understand the topic at hand. Yet for others it is a foundation from which pharmacists will be lifelong learners, aiming to communicate their knowledge to others.

Future practice competencies will need to not only address the knowledge of the profession, but also the qualities of what others consider consistent with being a "good pharmacist." The authors agree with Jungnickel, et al.[5] that tomorrow's pharmacists will consistently provide visible patient-centered and population–based care that improves medication therapy outcomes, and therefore will have a significant role in wellness and disease prevention activities.

> *Ninety-five percent (95%) of student pharmacists graduating in 2009 felt prepared to enter pharmacy practice.*
> *–AACP [6]*

Finally, on graduation, the outcomes of the curriculum should tie-in the vows taken in the *Oath of a Pharmacist* (Figure 6.1). Many schools begin the first week of classes for first year student pharmacists with an orientation that includes the oath. Should this oath be asked each year stressing the promise of a lifetime of service as a "good pharmacist?"

Figure 6.1. The Oath of the Pharmacist

I promise to devote myself to a lifetime of service to others through the profession of pharmacy. In fulfilling this vow:

I will consider the welfare of humanity and relief of suffering my primary concerns

I will apply my knowledge, experience, and skills to the best of my ability to assure optimal outcomes for my patients

I will respect and protect all personal and health information entrusted to me

I will accept the lifelong obligation to improve my professional knowledge and competence

I will hold myself and my colleagues to the highest principles of our profession's moral, ethical, and legal conduct

I will embrace and advocate changes that improve patient care

I will utilize my knowledge, skills, experiences, and values to prepare the next generation of pharmacists.

I take these vows voluntarily with the full realization of the responsibility with which I am entrusted by the public.

Revised 2009

TRAINING AND DEVELOPMENT

What are the goals that our profession has set for training and professional development? This is a difficult question to address, as the response depends on practice site, size of the organization, and the overall goals and objectives of the company, institution, or government agency that employs the trained pharmacist. Some look at professional development goals as a means to reach the minimal requirements of licensure, while others look at this as a means to grow personally and professionally.

For mentorship, preceptorship, and leadership development, some schools require preceptors to complete training. Does the training include the qualities of a "good pharmacist?" If it does, the next step will be to discover if these preceptors are applying the training and skills for visible patient-centered care. There is debate whether these characteristics or qualities can be taught. However, we hope that seeing the possibilities and providing the parallel learning in patient care provides an opportunity to at least be engaged in MTM and other clinical services.

LIFELONG LEARNING

Finally, a professional is expected to stay up-to-date on professional practice and research. This is a lifelong learning process that is based on the desire for knowledge and results in professional growth.

> *General separation is made between the pre-service preparatory years – when the foundation of competence are established and the later years of active practice – when increasing competence is a constantly tested performance.*
> *–Cyril Houle[7]*

Lifelong learning not only addresses the knowledge of the profession and how one can improve one's skills and competencies in knowledge, but also addresses the question of the delivery of this knowledge so that it can lead to innovation in practice.

Summary - "Providing quality, patient-centered care needs a knowledge base continuously expanded and updated."[8] All "good pharmacists" know this to be true. The complex professionalization process between thinking about becoming a pharmacist to a student pharmacist walking across the stage at graduation makes a novice into a professional. The faculty and preceptors guiding this professionalization process need to push the envelope and to mentor our future practitioners to be "good pharmacists."

Schools of pharmacy need to reconsider that IPPE and APPE experiential training is not just a check box on a form, but should be based on a clinical competency goal that is observed and evaluated by the preceptor.

Preceptors must also challenge student pharmacists to apply their didactic knowledge in every rotation and provide the understanding that pharmacists must tailor their counseling information for each patient by applying their clinical knowledge with genuine care for the patient.

Chapter Notes

1   Boyce, EG; Lawson, LA. "Preprofessional Curriculum in Preparation for the Physician of Pharmacy Education Programs. AACP Curricular Change Summit Supplement." *Am J Pharm Educ.* 2009;73 (8) article 155.

2   Accreditation Council for Pharmacy Education. Accreditation Standards and Guidelines for the Professional Program in Pharmacy Leading to the Physician of Pharmacy Degree. ACPE, Chicago Illinois. 2006 (Effective date July 1, 2007).

3   Understanding the Pathways of the Ph.D. Degree in Pharmaceutical Sciences, American Foundation of Pharmaceutical Education / American Association of Pharmaceutical Pharmacists, 2007; Unpublished document.

4   Personal Communication between William Kelly and a Disney World Representative. Orlando, FL., 2/25/10.

5   Jungnickel, PW; Kelly, WK; Hammer, DP; et al. "Addressing Competencies For the Future in the Professional Curriculum. AACP Curricular Change Summit Supplement." *Am J Pharm Educ.* 2009; 73(8) Article 156.

6   Graduating Pharmacy Student Survey Summary Report – 2009. American Association of Colleges of Pharmacy. Alexandria VA

7   Houle, CQ. *Continuing Learning in the Professions.* San Francisco: Jossey-Bass Publishers, 1980.

8   Burke, JN; Miller, WA; Spencer, AP; et al. "Clinical Pharmacist Competencies." *Pharmacotherapy.* 2008;28 (6):806-815

Chapter Seven

Am I a "Good Pharmacist?"

If you are a practicing pharmacist and need guidance on whether you are a "good pharmacist," then we encourage you to use the assessment tool below.

Before you begin the assessment, please agree to be honest so you can discover where you are on the road to maximizing your potential as a pharmacist. No one will see the results but you. Place a score (1 to 4) in the far right column after each question using the following scoring:

4 = always 3 = most of the time 2 = some of the time 1= never.

Question	Score
I TAKE AN INTEREST AND AM DIRECTLY INVOLVED (HAVE A CONSISTENT FACE-TO-FACE CONTACT) WITH PATIENTS	
MY ACTIONS SHOW I CARE ABOUT PATIENTS	
I USE MY KNOWLEDGE OF DRUGS AND DRUG THERAPY TO HELP PATIENTS MAKE THE BEST USE OF THEIR MEDICATION TO AVOID SUFFERING AND NEEDLESS EXPENSE	
I AM AVAILABLE, APPROACHABLE, AND ATTENTIVE TO PATIENT NEEDS	
I WORRY ABOUT CERTAIN PATIENTS AFTER I GO HOME	
I IDENTIFY, RESOLVE, PREVENT, AND REFER MEDICATION-RELATED PROBLEMS	
I AM FRIENDLY AND PUT FORTH EXTRA EFFORT FOR PATIENTS AND FELLOW HEALTH PROVIDERS	
I LISTEN CAREFULLY, COMMUNICATE WELL WITH PATIENTS, AND CHECK FOR UNDERSTANDING	
I CONSISTENTLY COUNSEL PATIENTS ABOUT THEIR MEDICATION	
I RECEIVE COMPLIMENTS FROM PATIENTS ABOUT THE CARE I PROVIDE	
Total Score	

Scoring:

35-40: You are a "good pharmacist"

25-34: You probably are a "good pharmacist"

16-24: You may need to make some changes in your practice to be a "good pharmacist"

0-15: You may need to make significant changes in your practice to be a "good pharmacist."

If you scored lower than you thought you would, it is possible: 1) you spend most of your time doing non-practitioner or administrative duties, 2) you have limited patient care contact, or 3) you have scored yourself too harshly (please review your answers and take the test again). This exercise is by no means a decisive indicator of being a "good pharmacist." Using this assessment tool is merely a starting point. You will also know if you are a "good pharmacist" by the positive comments you receive from patients and other health professionals.

Summary –By completing this self-assessment, you are taking your first step towards being a better pharmacist. But the road does not end here. It is up to you to take the next steps. The following chapter is designed to help.

Chapter Eight

Becoming a "Good Pharmacist"

In Chapter 6, we discussed the characteristics of what makes a "good pharmacist," and how to use these characteristics as criteria and ideals in the selection, education, and training of student pharmacists. In this chapter we offer suggestions on how a pharmacist, who is not yet a "good pharmacist," can become more patient-centered and "good." If you completed the self-assessment tool in the previous chapter and your score did not reflect where you want to be, this chapter will help you become a better pharmacist.

Challenges to Becoming a "Good Pharmacist"

There are several challenges to being a "good pharmacist." Here are a few:

Self-Image – The way you define your role as a pharmacist relates directly to your set of priorities when practicing pharmacy. For example, do you feel that your primary responsibility is to quickly and accurately dispense medication? Is it to produce prescription labels, and to count, measure and prepare medication? Is it to counsel patients about their medication? Is it to help patients in the OTC aisle of the pharmacy? Is it to help patients make the best use of their medication and to avoid suffering and needless expense? Answering these questions is the key to who you are as a pharmacist. The authors feel strongly that the correct answer to each of these questions is "yes."

Workload – Everyone experiences a heavy workload at times. It is not so much the workload, but how you handle it. Often we see pharmacists succumb to a heavy workload by becoming nothing but a "super pharmacy technician," performing all the technical functions of a pharmacist while ignoring the more patient-centered functions of the profession. When extremely busy, some pharmacists just want to get the "work out the door."

Not Enough Technician and Technology Support – We hear frequent complaints that some pharmacists do not have enough technician and technology support to help free time for more patient-centered care. While these complaints are frequently true, often they may be an excuse.

Employer or Supervisor Resistance – We acknowledge that some employers or supervisors may resist visible patient-centered care, and thus not allow pharmacists to use their skills in identifying, preventing, resolving, or referring medication-related problems. In our research we heard complaints such as: "They will not let us do it." The "they" may be a supervisor, pharmacy owner, or employer. It is disturbing if "they" is another pharmacist.

Lack of Clinical Skills – For sure, not all pharmacists have been trained clinically. However, a pharmacist should embrace the duty of lifelong learning, and no longer use their lack of original training as an excuse. There are ways for everyone to become more clinically competent.

Lack of Visible Patient-Centered Skills – Unlike clinical skills that may involve gaining new knowledge, visible patient-centered skills are intuitive, and can be learned quickly by just making yourself available to the patient and being friendly. Claiming a lack of these skills may be no more than a resistance to leaving one's comfort zone.

Steps to Becoming a Better Pharmacist

There are several steps a pharmacist can take to become a better pharmacist and strive to become a "good pharmacist."

Clarify Your Duties, Values, and Practice Plan – This is the most important step in becoming a better pharmacist. Is your first duty to your employer or to the patient? Is your primary responsibility to process the prescription or is it to provide visible patient-centered care? This is about your professional self-image and what's most important to you. Is it the medication? Is it trying to impress prescribers with your knowledge? Or, is it the patient?

Chelsea Baker, a 13 year-old from Plant City, Florida may be the best Little League pitcher in the country because of a knuckleball she mastered after learning the pitch from Joe Niekro, a major-league pitcher. In 2010, she pitched two perfect games, was profiled by ESPN, and approached by movie producers. The National Baseball Hall of Fame wanted her jersey. When asked what her secret was, her stepdad said "It starts in the heart."[1]

Do you have a heart for patients? If you do, are you meeting and talking with patients face-to-face about their medication, or are you hiding from patients saying you are too busy? Here a few short steps to clarify your values and practice plan:

Write a Tribute to Yourself as a Pharmacist – This tribute should state what you do well and which of your daily duties gives you the most pride.

Write a Credo – Start by writing "As a pharmacist I believe
……"

Evaluate Your Credo with Others – Test your credo with other
pharmacists and fellow workers. Even try it on your friends
and patients. Ask them: "What do you expect of me as a pharmacist?" and: "How can I help you the most?"

Build Your Practice Plan – This does not need to be elabo-
rate. It can be as simple as writing something like 'each day I
will meet face-to-face with at least five patients and help them
make the best use of their medication, and avoid suffering and
needless expense'. You may want to have a statement on learning new clinical knowledge and another one on learning new
clinical skills. How about meeting with physicians to develop a
collaborative practice arrangement (if permitted by state law)?
What about building opportunities for MTM on referral? A
roadmap is available to do this.[2]

A journey of a thousand miles begins with a single step
–Lao-tzu Chinese Philosopher (604 BC - 531 BC)

Taming the Workload Monster – Let us start with a question:
"Who is the best pharmacist? The one who can fill the most prescriptions or drug orders, or the one who makes sure all the work gets
done and still has time to meet face-to-face with patients?"

We hear pharmacists complaining of "too much work," yet
investigation often reveals that they are not using pharmacy technicians wisely or pushing for technology and automation. In regard
to the workload in traditional pharmacy, many pharmacists need to

see themselves more like a conductor, rather than a member of the orchestra.

Whose Job Is It? All pharmacists are recipients of an outstanding professional education, and therefore should not regress to technicians when they enter practice. However, this happens more than it should.

In community pharmacy practice, well-trained (and hopefully certified) pharmacy technicians should be performing all of the traditional and technical functions – data entry, preparing the medication, affixing the label, and ringing up the sale. If you are a community pharmacist, how much of your day is spent doing these technical functions? It should be very little.

Instead you should be: greeting each patient, accepting and clarifying the information on the prescription and asking about allergies. The pharmacist should be the one that clarifies all prescription issues with the prescriber and checks the accuracy of the medication label to be dispensed to the patient. But, it is also the pharmacist's function (not the technician's or clerk's function) to counsel the patient about their medication. If you are a community pharmacist, how often are you performing these professional functions? It should be most of the time.

Ideally, in the hospital or health-system pharmacy, pharmacy technicians should be the ones entering medication order information into the computer, and preparing and labeling the medication. If you are a hospital or health system pharmacist, how much of these technical functions are you performing every day? Hospital pharmacists should clarify orders with prescribers, and then check the data entry, the prepared medication, and labeling before it is dispensed to patients, then use the balance of the time having face-to-face contact with patients each day.

Heavy workload is rarely constant. In almost every pharmacy, time is available when workload slows. This is when you follow your practice plan and perform your visible patient-centered care, hopefully building towards intertwining it consistently throughout the ebb and flow of the normal work day.

Not Enough Technician and Technology Support – Despite our general observation that many pharmacists have to deal with insufficient technician and technology support, we also see cases where pharmacists are not using technicians or technology optimally. Not delegating work to technicians or avoiding the use of technology to improve efficiency and safety is a disservice to pharmacists and patients alike. Without correction, this problem becomes a supervisory issue that needs attention.

But, let us assume you are a pharmacist who uses technicians and technology optimally, how do you obtain more help so you can practice patient-centered care? Can you provide a business plan for more help in a community setting that underscores a return on the investment, showing that this will drive business through loyalty of patients based on the quality of the care you provide in your environment? Documenting your interactions and interventions will also help to support the need for greater help.

In the institution, can you document the increases in requests for information, not only by patients, but also by the other health care professionals you work with? Can you show how face-to-face interactions with patients in the hospital provides a better understanding of the medications and thus yield a better satisfaction with pharmacy services?

The first and perhaps most important question senior student pharmacists should ask potential employers is: "How much technician and technology support are you going to provide for me if I work for you?" rather than "how much are you going to pay me."

Overcoming Supervisor or Employer Resistance – "They will not let us do it." The "they" in this sentence is often illusive, not at all making clear who does not seem to be in favor of visible patient-centered or pharmaceutical care. Did someone (a supervisor, employer, or owner) actually say that to you, or are you supposing this is the case?

Several options exist to confront such perceived or actual resistance from superiors:

First, you can chat with the person directly. Are they resistant, partially resistant, indifferent, or supportive? You may need to explain why you want to practice visible patient-centered care, and discuss the employer benefits that will accrue. This would include patient loyalty that will follow you as an individual *and* the pharmacy or pharmacy department in a health system environment.

Second, do you need permission? As the saying goes, it may be easier to beg for forgiveness than it is to ask for permission. After all, there is a certain professional autonomy that comes with being a pharmacist. You should practice the way you feel is best for you and your patients. But, it needs to be ethical and legal, and all the work must get done in a reasonable time frame through time management and the appropriate use of pharmacy technicians.

Third, if you are not allowed to practice visible patient-centered care, you should consider finding a place where you will be allowed to do that.

Fourth, document your interventions and outcomes of your visible patient-centered care, and share the list with your supervisor every two weeks.

Supervisors should and often do appreciate concrete examples and suggestions for improving patient satisfaction and loyalty. This challenge will be discussed further in the next chapter – allowing pharmacists to be "good."

Acquiring Clinical Knowledge – The pharmacists we know are knowledgeable about the pharmacology and pharmacokinetics of the drugs they dispense, but some have not been trained clinically to understand rational therapeutics fully. How does a pharmacist in this latter category acquire the clinical knowledge to help patients? Here are six suggestions:

1. Learn something new each day about drug therapy. If you are not learning, you are going backwards. We have a duty to embrace lifelong learning.
2. Adopt a role model, and associate with other pharmacists who are helping patients make the best use of their medication and avoid suffering and needless expense.
3. Adopt at least one therapeutic category in which to develop superior expertise.
4. Adopt an attitude that you are not expected to know everything.
5. Don't be afraid to say "I don't know the answer to that question." But, quickly follow this by saying, "but I will

find out." Ask other pharmacists for help. Most importantly follow-up!

6 Read, read, and read. Register for e-mailed tables of contents from leading clinical journals. Regularly review the FDA's dedicated web pages for healthcare professionals that serve as a gateway to drug safety (http://www.fda.gov/Drugs/ResourcesForYou/HealthProfessionals/default.htm).

Share a subscription to the *Medical Letter* and the *Pharmacist Letter* with other pharmacists.

Acquiring Patient-Centered Skills – Being able to provide visible patient-centered care is not dependent on your educational degree, when you graduated, your age, whether you have done a residency or are board certified. It is about being attentive, being friendly and respectful, talking with patients about their medication, and showing interest.

Caring gains the patient's attention and cooperation. Once you have the patient's attention, you can work on medication timeliness, adherence, effectiveness, and safety.

Medication Timeliness – There are times when getting the first dose into the patient is important. For example, for a child with strep throat, administering the first dose (with a parent's permission) right in the pharmacy can be helpful to a quicker recovery. Helping to get the first dose of certain medications (an antibiotic for an ear infection) delivered quickly to the nursing unit for certain patients would also be helpful.

Medication Adherence – Of all health professionals, the pharmacist should have the primary responsibility for making sure the patient is compliant with taking the medication as prescribed. Pharmacists are in the best position to do that. The clinical and social gains of this practice are compelling, and therefore this is another scope of practice issue the profession needs to address.

Medication Effectiveness – Asking questions can often reveal whether the medication is actually working for a specific patient. Establishing baseline goals (like the number of seizures a month) with the patient serves as a benchmark. In community pharmacy, therapeutic goals can be set with the patient at the medication counseling step during the original dispensing. Factors interfering with effectiveness can be shared with the prescriber.

Medication Safety – Rather than waiting for a patient to volunteer or complain about a side or adverse effect, it is better to ask the patient.

In community pharmacy, the best time to check on medication effectiveness and safety is during the first refill. The key questions are: "How is the medication working for you," and "Are you experiencing any difficulties with this medication?" These questions are also valid for pharmacists to ask patients in organized health care settings, shortly after the medication has been prescribed. This gets the pharmacist into the patient's room and is visible patient-centered care.

Practice, Practice, Practice – The important step is to start, then continue to work at delivering patient-centered care. You will get better and better with time until it is routine, and you will wonder why you did not do this earlier. Make a habit of finding medication-related problems in patients: dose too high, dose too low, unnecessary therapy, use of a wrong drug, an untreated problem, not receiving the drug or poor adherence, or experiencing an adverse drug event.

Set a Goal for Seeing Patients Daily – As mentioned earlier, establishing a goal, such as meeting face-to-face with at least five patients every day, helps motivate you to get into the visible patient-centered groove. Five patients a day does not sound like much, but think about it – five patients a day is 25 a week, and over 1200 a year. Just think what would happen if every practicing pharmacist did that! Think what could happen if you went about interacting with one patient every hour you are working – that would be 40 patients each week (given a 40 hour work week) and more than 2000 patients a year.

Most important, keep thinking about what it will feel like to practice as a clinically competent, patient-centered pharmacist – a "good pharmacist."

Why Should I Do This?

Every group has its mercenaries. You might ask: "Why should I do this?" or "What is in it for me?" Such questions lead back to the past as to why you went into pharmacy in the first place while they also have future ramifications for admission questions asked by pharmacy schools.

Here are six possible answers to the question: "What is in it for me?" There are more than six answers, but we feel these are the main ones.

Satisfaction with Seeing Patients Improve – Seeing patients get better, either as a matter of course or because of something you did, may provide satisfaction. Isn't this the reason you went into pharmacy?

Job Satisfaction – The "good pharmacists" we interviewed agreed unanimously that their visible patient-centered care resulted in satisfaction that they were making a difference in patients' lives and they loved what they were doing. As encouragement, please go back and read these comments in Chapter 4 – What "Good Pharmacists Tell Us."

Positive Patient Feedback – When you practice visible patient-centered care, you will receive positive feedback and rewarding comments from patients. It is a given. Patients will tell you they like what you were able to do for them, and some may even pass this on to your supervisor. Such positive feedback should also be documented by the pharmacist.

Patient Loyalty – Patients who receive patient-centered care from a pharmacist will often seek out that pharmacist for future care. What better compliment is there than that? Pharmacy owners and employers will benefit because patients will remain loyal to the pharmacy where you practice. New patients will return for more patient-centered care. In fact they will probably tell friends and family about "their pharmacist" the way people tell others about "their doctor." That drives more patients to you and your business improves.

It Helps Improve Respect for the Profession – By providing visible patient-centered care, you will help change the public's perception of pharmacy from a product-focused profession to a patient-focused profession.

It Will Help Pharmacists Receive Reimbursement for Cognitive Services – The profession has a long standing dream to be recognized for improving patient outcomes. Receiving reimbursement for our clinical contributions will satisfy this goal. Each pharmacist, providing visible patient-centered care, one patient at a time, will make this dream a reality. But, this will only happen if such interventions are documented over time in a systematic fashion. Pharmacists can show their influence on enhanced patient outcomes by providing timely feedback about the effects of drug therapy to prescribers.

> *A clinical pharmacy practice brings its own rewards to the pharmacist. To be an expert in the clinical use of drugs presents a lifelong challenge of learning and self study. It brings professional respect from physicians and nurses and places the pharmacist in the mainstream of caring and healing. A career in clinical pharmacy is an open-ended opportunity for those who seek its rewards.[3]*
> *–William E. Smith*

Summary – Pharmacists who are not yet providing visible patient-centered care, and therefore are not yet "good pharmacists," can become one by: 1) realizing the benefits of practicing this way, 2) making visible patient-centered care their primary responsibility, 3) learning clinical and patient-centered skills, 4) meeting some patients face-to-face daily, and 5) preventing, identifying, resolving, or referring medication-related problems in their patients. The rewards for doing so are the most satisfying the profession has to offer.

Chapter Notes

1 Wilmath, K. "13 Years Old, Already in Cooperstown." Page 1-A. *St. Petersburg Times.* August 12, 2010.
2 Smith, M; Bates, DW; Bodenheimer, T; et al. "Why Pharmacists Belong in the Medical Home." *Health Affairs.* 2010;29(5):906-913.
3 Smith, WE. "Clinical Pharmacy in the 1980s. Whitney Award Address." *Am J Hosp Pharm.* 1983; 40:223-9

Chapter Nine

Allowing Pharmacists to be "Good"

Are there challenges that prevent or hinder a pharmacist from being a "good pharmacist?" Of course, just as there are challenges to performing any service or the ability to learn the knowledge of the profession. Our concern is focused on looking at the positive ways to overcome barriers, be they self-created, environmental, or external to the profession, and allowing all pharmacists to practice in a visible patient-centered clinical model.

Challenges that keep pharmacists from being good may exist in the environment (physical or policy), and may come from employers, supervisors, and support staff. We will analyze a few of these areas. However, a pharmacist seeking to be a "good pharmacist" overcomes these challenges no matter what.

Community Pharmacists

Community pharmacists have an excellent opportunity to conduct basic preliminary health assessments of patients. Quick evaluation of symptoms, laboratory values, and other services such as point of care testing, can be helpful in directing a patient's therapy, especially as the community pharmacist's role in visible patient-centered care continues to expand. Services such as medication therapy management (MTM), health screenings, first refill assessment, pharmacist administered immunizations, and other clinical-based disease state management services continue to expand the role and patient responsibilities of the individual community based practitioner. Pharmacists not only address these clinical services from a disease perspective but also need to be knowledgeable about nutrition, OTC's, health and wellness, so they can provide information at the point of care and take preventive measures.

As mentioned earlier, a pharmacist can provide these types of services by going through the checklist, or they can engage with the patient, provide a tailored service while being attentive and caring. The American Pharmacists Association (APhA) Career Pathway Evaluation Program for Pharmacy Professionals suggests that more than 50% of community based respondents consider patient care and contact as one of the most satisfying roles in the profession.[1]

Ideal community practice, be it in chain, independent, or other types of pharmacies, is directly associated with patient counseling and visible patient-centered care. In addition, most community pharmacists have good relationships with other health professionals in their communities. Pharmacists have an important role in keeping open communication with other health care providers about the medication therapy of patients, and alerting the prescriber to drug therapy problems.

Community practice leadership can be characterized by possessing vision and initiative - vision to guide an individual or organization to a goal, and initiative to take the steps necessary to reach that goal. These skills are often critical parts of personal career development and the qualities, characteristics and habits of the "good pharmacist."

On-the-job experience provides significant opportunities for developing leadership skills for community based pharmacists. This is critical, as pharmacists must decide and provide direction to support staff throughout the day. A pharmacist's ability to lead by example offers visual cues to others around them. The ability to gain the support, cooperation, and loyalty of co-workers or employees is important for the success of patient-centered care because it can take time away from other roles and responsibilities.

To adopt a visible patient-centered focus in community pharmacy, individuals must engage in the lifelong curricula discussed earlier. Lifelong learning may not take up much time, but is a necessary part of being a practicing community pharmacist. The environment can allow a pharmacist to be "good," but getting there takes work, dedication, understanding and the willingness to get all parties on the same page, moving forward.

HOSPITALS AND HEALTH-SYSTEM PHARMACISTS

Unlike community pharmacists who work with the public and their patients, hospital and health-system pharmacists work with other health care professionals, specifically nurses and physicians, physician assistants and nurse practitioners. In addition, greater opportunity exists to interact with many specialty caregivers in obstetrics, nutrition, oncology, transplant, surgery, infectious disease, pediatrics, geriatrics, nuclear pharmacy or other specialty areas.

In some health systems, however, opportunities exist for pharmacists to see patients by rounding with prescribers and nurses or when the pharmacist works in an outpatient clinic where they may have responsibility for direct visible patient-centered care. Pharmacists have the opportunity to interview patients for medications at admissions or discharge and any point between, when medication is added, changed or stopped. The APhA Career Pathway Evaluation Program for Pharmacy Professionals suggests that twenty-five percent of a hospital or health-system staff pharmacist's time is spent on patient care services.[1] But, does face-to-face contact occur with patients?

Professional and leadership development is different in the hospital or health-system setting. More layers or tiers of positions with different leadership roles are available. Examples include the number of directors (assistant, associate, etc.) that are needed based on the size of the institution. In the hospital or health-system, the support for the qualities of a "good pharmacist" will differ based on the hospital or health-system, size of the organization, and the way the pharmacy department implements visible patient-centered care.

A tertiary university based hospital provides a different type of support of the pharmacist's role. We see specialists in specific disease state areas (HIV, infectious disease, diabetes, etc.). In addition, one must consider those frontline hospital and health system pharmacists, who work in inpatient satellite pharmacies and have many opportunities to interact directly with patients. This is in contrast to a small rural community based hospital, which may require more diverse general knowledge based specialists.

With the varying and ever changing conditions and treatments a pharmacist faces in a hospital or health-system, staff and clinical pharmacists must continually keep up with new research and therapy regimens. The hospital or health-system is a natural place for lifelong learning, adding to one's knowledge set. Hospital and health-system pharmacists look at lifelong learning as a continual process as the patients treated by a hospital or health-system pharmacist typically have more complicated conditions than those in an ambulatory setting.

As with community settings, hospitals and health-systems can allow a pharmacist to be "good" – however, it takes the same work, dedication, and understanding to get all parties on the same page to move forward. The health issues associated with being a hospital or health-system patient can be different from that of an ambulatory patient.

EMPLOYEE AND EMPLOYER

For a pharmacist to be a "good pharmacist," the pharmacist and the employer (even when self-employed) must work together. It is a directive that a pharmacist must have within them – a commitment that provides the drive and passion to provide high quality visible patient-centered care. Even if an employer supports the direct patient care role and responsibility of the pharmacist, the individual pharmacist must deliver on the goals and objectives of this model.

Even with that emphasis, the employer provides the staffing, time, and assessment tools that address the current and future visible patient-centered roles of pharmacists. However, even if an individual has the drive, characteristics, qualities, and values discussed, an environment that does not support or promote pharmaceutical care can hinder, and even squelch the chance that this role and responsibility will be met. Problems can develop if the stated goals are narrowly focused and do not provide a visible patient-centered care model, including recognizing those who foster and promote these activities. Management may not appreciate when a pharmacist has to let the workload wait while she or he prevents harm or promotes good. In fact, management may assume that pharmacists will do that regardless of managerial pressure for productivity.

> *Although we've been educated as professionals and have maintained our competence, we have essentially no control over how we practice our profession. The control rests in the hands of our employers. Those employers, even those who are pharmacists, seem bound by a traditional concept of the role of the pharmacist.*[2]
> —William A. Zellmer

However, managers need to be careful when they preempt the professional judgment of their pharmacists. The environment and employer who hinders the "good pharmacist" from practicing at a level and quality of care all patients want, need, and deserve is doing a disservice to the "good pharmacist" and to their patients. However, we have seen some employers support the expanding role of a pharmacist by providing the opportunities, infrastructure, and recognition for those who provide patient-centered care. It would help if corporate pharmacies would use more than the primary metric of 'number of prescriptions dispensed a day,' and expand to 'number of patients counseled a day,' or 'number of patients seen face-to-face a day.'

A Word on Professional Autonomy

It must be remembered that the functions of the profession are not necessarily those of the institutional structure that house it. We need pharmacists who are "in, but not of" their institutions, whose allegiance to the core values of the profession (and their patients) makes them resist the institutional diminishment of those values.[3]

We are afraid that unless pharmacists muster the courage to exercise more professional autonomy, there is not much hope of nurturing more "good pharmacists." We feel this is a critical topic that needs immediate discussion and action within the profession.

> *How do I stay close to the passions and commitments that took me into this work – challenging myself, my colleagues, and my institution to keep faith with this profession's deepest values?*[3]
>
> *–Parker J. Palmer*

PROFESSIONAL ASSOCIATIONS

Perhaps the groups trying the hardest to allow pharmacists to be "good" are professional pharmacy associations. These can be local, state, national, or international. For most associations, the goal is to drive the profession to greater heights. However, at times this can also be at odds with allowing a pharmacist to be "good." One may ask how an association can be supportive and yet, unsupportive?

The professional associations provide the education for pharmacists to continue lifelong learning, they advocate for state and federal legislation that supports (or hinders) the pharmacist, they provide opportunities for leadership roles, and they anticipate the future. However, the level of the education and its ultimate impact to the practice site may be questionable. While associations mostly provide level one (introductory) education, level three (advanced) education is what is needed most. In addition, associations should also incorporate examples and cases that provide insight into the methods of a "good pharmacist" in applying the knowledge presented.

In contrast, professional associations are driven by membership who at times may find a vocal few who drive the profession in a direction that may not support or allow a pharmacist to be "good." As an example, a group may be vocal about the importance of credentialing within the profession without thought to the impact this will or will not have on providing opportunities for all pharmacists to practice as "good pharmacists." These groups use their own narrow definitions of what they consider to be "good." This is not to say the role that a small few play does not have its place. On the contrary, it was small groups that began to look at driving clinical roles for pharmacists, for MTM services, for cognitive skills reimbursement, and for change.

If it were not for a few vocal pharmacists who moved toward pharmacist administered immunizations, we would not be where we are today in providing immunizations and vaccines across the US to the patients and the communities we serve. The associations are directive groups that push for all pharmacists to be "good pharmacists," but need more consistency and professional unity in doing so.

PATIENTS

In some types of business, three words are the key to success – location, location, location. In pharmacy we may need to think about a mantra of three words to address visible patient-centered success – patients, patients, patients. Patients have the final say if a pharmacist delivers on all or any of the issues discussed. The patient can reject the offer, not listen, not care, feel this is not the pharmacists' role, or openly accept the information to make informed decisions in collaboration with the pharmacist and other health care team members.

So how do we get patients to allow us to be "good?" It has been a struggle for years to have anyone outside the profession (and a few in the profession as well) to understand the patient-centered role and responsibilities of the pharmacist. We must continue to rely on individual pharmacists to display the characteristics of a "good pharmacist" to patients. Even one by one, patients who have had the opportunity to work with a "good pharmacist" will spread the word.

We are aware of patients who look to the pharmacist for advice on many healthcare issues and consider these pharmacists "good pharmacists." We are aware of patients who travel past more "convenient" pharmacies to seek out a "good pharmacist." We are aware of patients that will call specific pharmacies for medication information (even if they receive the medication from a competitor), because all the pharmacists at that location are "good pharmacists."

Most importantly, we are aware of patients who will ask for a certain pharmacist because they trust that pharmacist, and know the pharmacist is looking out for their welfare. These patients know the pharmacist is taking full responsibility for their medication therapy management and have a positive experience with a "good pharmacist."

Yes, just one pharmacist can make a difference!

Summary – The environment (physical or policy), employers, supervisors, support staff, and others can inhibit a pharmacist from being "good." However, pharmacists need to push forward to be a "good pharmacist" despite these challenges.

Chapter Notes

1 APhA Career Pathway Evaluation Program. http://www. pharmacist.com/AM/Template.cfm?Section=Pathways Program&Template=/CM/ContentDisplay. cfm&ContentID=12183. Accessed April 21, 2010.

2 Zellmer, WA. "Dear Colleague. The Conscience of a Pharmacist." *American Society of Health-System Pharmacists.* Bethesda. 2002. Pages 145-147

3 Palmer, PJ. "A New Professional: The Aims of Education Revisited." *Change – The Magazine of Higher Education.* November – December, 2007. www.changemag.org/Archives/ Back%20Issues/November-December%202007/full-new-professional.html. Accessed 6/14/10.

Chapter Ten

If Most Pharmacists Were "Good Pharmacists"

*Most pharmacists are well trained, honest, hardworking profes-*sionals. Most of the ones we know take their professional roles seriously and try to follow the laws, regulations, standards, ethics, and professional traditions. Some of these pharmacists are also "good pharmacists" using the definition provided in this book.

How many "good pharmacists" are there? No one knows the answer to this compelling question, but we suspect it is a minority. We are confident that most pharmacist specialists certified by the Board of Pharmacy Specialties (BPS), and those who are credentialed as a Certified Geriatric Pharmacist (CGP), practice visible patient-centered care, but one need not be certified to be a "good pharmacist." However, the recent approval of ambulatory care pharmacy as a specialty by BPS may provide stimulus to a large number of pharmacists to practice in a visible patient-centered way. Similarly, the expanded MTM requirements under Medicare Part D will likely influence pharmacists who set priorities for patient-centered care to aim for the CGP credential.[1]

All pharmacists are knowledgeable (at least about the medications patients take), which is an unanimous characteristic of a "good pharmacist." Therefore, knowledge alone cannot be the distinguishing quality of the "good pharmacist. Instead, it is most likely providing visible patient-centered care. The main ingredient of providing visible patient-centered is caring. In turn, caring is the main feature of pharmaceutical care.

Do most pharmacists practice visible patient-centered care and display caring behavior towards patients? We think many do, but most are still not positioned to care. They may hide behind the prescription counter and the four walls of a hospital or health-system pharmacy. They rarely, if ever, interact with patients. They make excuses by saying they have too many prescriptions or drug orders. Yet, many of these same pharmacists are not using pharmacy technicians properly, not demanding only the use of certified technicians, not insisting on automation that can improve safety and liberate them to be with patients.

> *Vision with action is a dream. Action without vision is simply passing time. Action with vision is making a positive difference.*
> *–Joel Barker Independent Scholar & Futurist*

Does this mean that after 25 years, pharmaceutical care has failed? We must keep in mind that pharmacy practice is changing, and despite our desire, change does not take place overnight, but it can take place.[2] We must put forth more effort to put more visible patient-centered care into our profession. We need more backbone to stand up and say to those who employ us – we MUST practice our profession in a patient-centered fashion. Perhaps we need more vision. If so, here it is: *What would happen if most pharmacists were "good pharmacists?"*

THE IMPACT ON PATIENTS

If most pharmacists were "good pharmacists," patients would better understand and appreciate what a "good pharmacist" can provide. They would know they have a friend and trusted professional interested in their welfare. Patients would come to expect more from pharmacists. More pharmacist interaction with patients will bring about safer and more effective drug therapy and avoid patient suffering and economic waste – in short, better patient outcomes. Patients would look to their pharmacist for health and wellness information and implement their recommendations.

THE IMPACT ON OTHER HEALTH PROFESSIONALS

If most pharmacists were "good pharmacists," other health professionals – especially physicians and nurses – would have even more respect for us. Displaying a true caring attitude would help dissolve turf issues between providers. Physicians would respect us for our expertise in drug therapy and rely on us more. More respect will bring higher expectations – more opportunity to serve – better outcomes. Patients need teamwork. Our intelligence is no longer enough.

THE IMPACT ON EMPLOYERS

If most pharmacists were "good pharmacists," those who employ and supervise pharmacists would know the profession considers patients its number one concern; not the speed of the service we provide; not the number of prescriptions we process in an hour; and not profit from selling a product. The profession should display a caring attitude, concern for safety, and provide quality drug therapy. The only way to do that successfully is with liberal patient contact.

The profession should never tolerate outside pressure to practice a certain way or allow control by those outside the profession. We should always stand up and "mind the gap" for patients.

As employee pharmacists, we need to show employers how practicing as "good pharmacists" benefits the company or institution. Patients love "good pharmacists," are loyal to them, and want more of what "good pharmacists" provide. Employers who hire only "good pharmacists" and allow these pharmacists to be good will be rewarded. How? With an endless supply of "good pharmacists," high pharmacist retention rates, more business, and happier, more loyal customers. While some employers have shifted their thoughts to hiring pharmacists who are interested in a patient care model, other employers will need to change their practice from hiring "whatever pharmacist" to hiring only "good pharmacists."

THE IMPACT ON PHARMACISTS

If most pharmacists were "good pharmacists," there would be more job satisfaction. We base this hypothesis on the anecdotal information gathered when we interviewed the eleven pharmacists for Chapter 4. Suggestions exist that "good pharmacists" continually nurture close relationships with patients, and give patients their full measure of care. These patients often provide positive feedback to the pharmacist. We also believe that practicing like a "good pharmacist" produces the respect most pharmacists crave from patients, other health providers, and the media.

THE IMPACT ON THE PROFESSION

If most pharmacists were "good pharmacists," it would direct our professional destiny – a destiny with three possible outcomes:

Deprofessionalization – In this outcome, the profession allows those outside the profession to further reduce performance to the lowest common denominator. Most pharmacists hide behind their counters or in the health-system pharmacy and practice more like super technicians than visible patient-centered pharmacists. Patients view our role solely as dispensers of medication. Payers see us as overpaid and an unnecessary part of delivering medication to patients. Most patients obtain their medication from ATM-type machines found in physicians' offices. The profession moves backwards.

Business As Usual – Under this outcome, "good pharmacists" make patients the center of their practice, but most pharmacists practice pharmacy without much interaction with patients. The emphasis is on processing prescriptions and drug orders with some talk of improving medication safety, but with little progress made. The profession cannot move forward.

A True Visible Patient-Centered Clinical Profession – In this outcome, the dream of universal clinical pharmacy services is fulfilled.[3] Pharmacists are recognized for their expertise in medication and medication therapy, and their caring attitude towards patients. The profession reaches its full potential as a true clinical profession. Pharmacists receive reimbursement for clinical contributions that improve patient outcomes and for preventing serious medication misadventures. Respect for pharmacists soars to an all-time high.

> *"To every man there openeth*
> *A way and ways and a way;*
> *The high soul treads the high way,*
> *And the low soul gropes the low,*

And in between on the misty flats,
The rest draft to and fro."

–John Oxenham, English Poet (1852-1941)

CREATING THE TIPPING POINT

Pharmaceutical care is, at best, sputtering along and in need of a catalyst to reach a tipping point.[4] We are doubtful recent healthcare reform will provide the necessary stimulus to affect major change in the profession. The change needs to come from within. Therefore, the profession should identify the catalyst that will help most pharmacists become "good pharmacists." Our recommendation is that we not wait too long.

Summary – Seeking a catalyst and tipping point for most pharmacists to be "good pharmacists" may be the only viable strategy for the profession to fulfill its destiny as a true patient-centered clinical profession.

Chapter Notes

1   Smith, M; Bates, DW; Bodenheimer, T; et al. "Why Pharmacists Belong in the Medical Home." *Health affairs.* 2010; 29(%): 906-913.

2   Abramowitz, PA. "The Evolution and Metamorphosis of the Pharmacy Practice Model. The 2009 Harvey A.K. Whitney Address." *Am J Health-Syst Pharm.* 2009; 66: 1437-1446.

3   Hepler, CD. "A Dream Deferred. The 2010 Harvey AK Whitney Address." *The Am. Soc. Health-Sys Pharmacists Annual Meeting.* Tampa, FL June 8, 2010.

4   Gladwell, Malcolm. *The Tipping Point.* Boston: Little Brown and Company, 2002.

Afterword

We realize fully our investigation of the "good pharmacist" is based on limited information, and therefore generates a hypothesis. We will continue to study the idea and welcome others to either confirm or dispute our findings.

We also know that just because one person thinks a pharmacist is a "good pharmacist" does not necessarily make it true. This highlights the nature and limitation of qualitative research, the results of which produce a hypothesis that is either accepted or rejected by more objective methods.

We acknowledge there are many good pharmacists who work in administrative positions that do not lend themselves to direct patient care. We do not wish to slight them in any way. However, Directors of Pharmacy, Pharmacy Managers, and Pharmacy Supervisors in organized health care settings and in corporate pharmacies should get out of their offices to see how well their pharmacists are performing visible patient-centered care.

Identifying and removing barriers to this practice are in the best interest of your organization and patients.

Although this book is intended for pharmacy educators, practicing pharmacists, student pharmacists, and those who manage pharmacies and pharmacists, any pharmacist and perhaps other health care providers and patients will benefit from reading it.

Major Recommendations

Recommendation	Who	Chapter	Page
DESIGN AN OUTCOME-BASED CURRICULUM BASED ON WHAT MAKES A "GOOD PHARMACIST."	PHARMACY FACULTY	1 6	29 90
INVESTIGATE HOW TO MOTIVATE PHARMACISTS TO CARE ABOUT PATIENTS.	PROFESSION	3	48
INCLUDE OTC COUNSELING IN THE SCOPE OF PRACTICE.	PROFESSION	3	52
INVESTIGATE WHY THE PUBLIC TRUSTS PHARMACISTS AND CONSIDER INCORPORATING IMPORTANT FINDINGS INTO EDUCATION, TRAINING, AND THE SCOPE OF PRACTICE.	PROFESSION	5	74
INVESTIGATE WAYS IN COMMUNITY PHARMACY PRACTICE THAT ALLOW PATIENTS TO READILY DISTINGUISH THE PHARMACIST FROM OTHER EMPLOYEES IN THE PHARMACY.	PROFESSIONAL ASSOCIATIONS	5	76
INVESTIGATE MAKING OR STRENGTHENING COUNSELING A PATIENT ABOUT THEIR MEDICATION A SCOPE OF PRACTICE ISSUE.	PROFESSION	3	52
TAILOR THE ADMISSIONS PROCESS OF A SCHOOL OF PHARMACY TO ATTRACT STUDENT PHARMACISTS WHO WILL BE ABLE TO GAIN AND APPLY THE KNOWLEDGE OF THE PROFESSION, SEEK LEADERSHIP ROLES, AND BY EXAMPLE BE "GOOD PHARMACISTS." HOW MUCH WEIGHT IS GIVEN TO THE PATIENT-CENTERED QUALITIES VS. A GPA?	PHARMACY FACULTY	6	86
DESIGN THE HIRING PROCESS TO INCLUDE QUESTIONS ABOUT QUALITIES AND CHARACTERISTICS OF HOW THE APPLICANT WILL PRACTICE WITHIN THE PROFESSION.	HIRING MANAGERS	1 6 10	30 88 134
MOVE TOWARD A CE PROCESS THAT PROVIDES TRAINING ABOUT BEING A "GOOD PHARMACIST" AND PRACTICAL DEMONSTRATIONS OF HOW THIS CAN BE INCORPORATED INTO EVERY DAY PRACTICE.	PROVIDERS OF PHARMACY CE	6	94

BASE PRECEPTOR SELECTION AND EVALUATION ON BROADER NEEDS IN THE EXPERIENTIAL SITES – GOING PAST THE KNOWLEDGE AND APPLICATION CHECK LIST TO ACTUAL PRACTICE ENVIRONMENT THAT SUPPORTS "GOOD PHARMACISTS."	EXPERIENTIAL EDUCATORS	1 6	29 91
REVIEW AND DETERMINE IF YOU EDUCATE AND PRACTICE ACCORDING TO THE OATH OF A PHARMACIST.	PHARMACY FACULTY, PHARMACISTS	6	92
SUPPORT THE PRACTICE AND CHARACTERISTICS OF "GOOD PHARMACISTS."	MANAGERS AND SUPERVISORS	6	124
TAKE THE SURVEY – ARE YOU A "GOOD PHARMACIST?"	PHARMACISTS	7	99
DEVELOP A STANDARD OF PRACTICE THAT ONLY CERTIFIED PHARMACY TECHNICIANS BE USED IN PHARMACIES.	PROFESSION	3	51
INVESTIGATE MAKING CHECKING MEDICATION ADHERENCE A NECESSARY PART OF THE PRESCRIPTION REVIEW AND PROCESSING.	PROFESSION	8	111
INVESTIGATE AND MAKE RECOMMENDATIONS CONCERNING PROFESSIONAL AUTONOMY IN PHARMACY.	PROFESSION	9	124

Appendix

Some Good Pharmacists

The following is a list of pharmacists who are considered to be "good pharmacists" as of the printing of this book. To nominate a pharmacist for future editions, either: 1) use the form that follows and mail or fax it to the authors, or 2) go to: www.thegoodpharmacist. com to complete a short online survey.

Angie – Durham, NC

Eldon Armstrong – Columbia, SC

Lenny Arteaga – Miami, FL

Joseph Barone – Piscataway, NJ

Peter Barron – Dunedin, New Zealand

CA Bond – Amarillo, TX[1]

Bob Brashear – Iverness, FL

Gerald Briggs – Huntington Beach, CA

Bruce Broadrick – Dalton, GA

Jake Brown – Atlanta, GA[1]

Steve Caddick – Tampa, FL

Alex Cardoni – Ellington, CT

Henry Cohen – Brooklyn, NY

Michael Cohen – Philadelphia, PA

Nancy Connors - Unknown

Brad Cooper – Erie, PA[2]

Michael Cotugno – Boston, MA
Dave – Chapel Hill, NC
Steven Dendiak – Atlanta, GA[1]
James DuBe – Omaho, NE
Cecily DiPiro – Charleston, SC
Maduekwe Elechukwu – Paortharcourt, Nigeria
Ed Elzarian – Hampton, VA
Joe Farins – Soap Lake, WA
Elisha Guadalupe – Nashville, TN
Kenneth Gillman – Bronx, NY
Jennifer Howard – Iowa City, IA
Mr. Jackson – Anderson, IN
Les Jameson – Chicago, IL
Dr. Jones – Khartoum, Sudan
Ira Katz – Atlanta, GA
Kellynna – Metaire, LA
Ken – Orlando, FL
Kayla Kosel – Seattle, WA
Steve Kutner – Bethesda, MD
Gary Lang – New Bern, NC
John M. – Dunedin, FL
Mike Madelon – Madison, WI
Richard Manny – Tampa, FL
Ray Marcrom – Manchester, TN
Kim Martin – Boise, ID
Melissa Somma McGiveny – Pittsburgh, PA
Thomas McGregor – Waukesha, WI[1]

Mike – Sauk Rapids, MN

Douglas Miller – O'Fallon, MO

Tenny Moss – Florence, SC

Richard Manny – Tampa, FL

Louis Mundy – Tyrone, GA

Sheila Neiman – Brooklyn, NY

Richard Owensy – Morganton, NC

Anna Parmenter – Hickory, NC[2]

Linette Pho – Chicago, IL

Bob Poole – Marietta, GA[1]

Jennifer Puno – Tacloban, Phillipines

Michael Romano – Pittsburgh, PA

Susan Rosendahl – Erie, PA

Zack Rutkowski – Detroit, MI

Kevin Scarlett – Newport, NH

Rick Schnatz – Rockville, MD

Renee Smith – Valdosta, GA

Elliott Sogol – Durham, NC[2]

Suellyn Sorensen – Indianapolis, IN

Jerry Storm – Peoria, IL

Lynda Thomson – Philadelphia, PA

Samuel Toggas – York, PA

Denise Toyer – Rockville, MD

Francis Unrein – Plainville, KS

Bob VanAntwerp – Louisville, KY[1]

April Vanis – Marietta, GA

Wayne – Houston, TX

Fred Wenk – Ann Arbor, MI

Robert Weber – Pittsburgh, PA

Rachel Wolfberg – Chicago, IL

Zaineb – Kuwait City, Kuwait

Zala – Compton, CA

[1] *deceased*

[2] *nominated more than once*

Note: *28 pharmacists were nominated where the person doing the nominating could not remember the name of the pharmacist.*

Contributors

The following is a list of those who nominated someone as a "good pharmacist" and wanted to be listed.

Ralph Allen, MD

Fred Bender, Pharm.D.

Steve Belknap, MD

Richard Bertin, Ph.D.

Richard Blum, MD

Wanda Bocanegra, RN

William Brereton, MD

Barbara Brown

Dan Buffington, Pharm.D.

Steven Caddick, Pharm.D.

Christin Carlin, RN

Tina Castro

Maureen Cahill, RN

Ifegbo Chisom, RPh

Jim Clark

Daniel Cobaugh, Pharm.D.

Kevin Colgan, RPh

Mike Flagstad, MS

Laurie Forrester, Pharm.D.

Carla Frye, Pharm.D.

Michael Giddings

Zachary Hannan, MS

Marybeth Harwick

Fran Hitchcock, RN

Judith Jones, MD, Ph.D.

Ira Katz, RPh

Patrick Kavanaugh

Nadir Kheir, Pharm.D.

Walter Kraf, MD

Bruce Laingen

Rafaela Lee, RPh

Sibley Leow

John Malone

Denise Mason

Nitu Matthew

James O'Donnell, Pharm.D.

Raphael Orenstein, MD

Jessi Owensby

Linda Paterniti, RPh

Jenny Pegg

Marjorie Phillips, RPh

James Ray, Pharm.D.

Riham, RPh

Gordon Schiff, MD

Rick Schnatz, Pharm.D.

Andy Shaw, Pharm.D.

William Smith, Ph.D., Pharm.D.

Elliott Sogol, Ph.D.

Whitney Sogol

Victoria Steelman, RN

Mark Sullivan, Pharm.D.

Sue Thomson, RN

Thomas Thompson, RPh

Fran Todd

Cliff Walker, Pharm.D.

Ida Williams, RN

Shu Yu Zhang

Nominate a Good Pharmacist

To nominate a practitioner pharmacist you feel is or was a "good pharmacist" you can do so online here: http://tinyurl.com/2d5q3co

Or you can email, FAX, or mail your nomination to:

> William N. Kelly
> 2147 Warwick Drive Oldsmar, Florida 34677
> E-MAIL: wnkelly@earthlink.net
> FAX: (727) 786-3424

Please include an example of how the named pharmacist demonstrated the characteristics of a "good pharmacist" along with the following data:

a Nominee's name
b Three adjectives (SINGLE WORDS), in order of importance, that describe the person you nominate as a "good pharmacist."
c Is this pharmacist still living? If yes, please provide his or her contact information if known.

Do you grant William N. Kelly and Elliott M. Sogol permission to use the information provided with the understanding that some, none, or all the information may be published?

Do you want your name listed as a contributor if this information is published? Please provide the following:

> Your name and title or degrees
> Your email address
> Your gender and age range: (<36 36-49 50-65 >65)

Thank you for contributing!

Index

Other Books by the Authors

William N. Kelly

Pharmacy: What It Is and How It Works. Taylor and Francis. Boca Raton, FL. 2002, 2007, 2011.

Prescribed Medication and the Public Health – Laying the Foundation for Risk Reduction. Pharmaceutical Products Press, now Taylor and Francis. Boca Raton, FL. 2006.

Elliott M. Sogol

Glaxo Pathway Evaluation Program for Medical Professionals: Specialty Profiles, Editor, Third Edition, Glaxo Wellcome Inc., Research Triangle Park, NC. 1996.

Glaxo Pathway Evaluation Program for Pharmacy Professionals: Career Option Profiles, Editor, Second Edition, Glaxo Inc., Research Triangle Park, NC. 1993.

Glaxo Pathway Evaluation Program for Medical Professionals: Specialty Profiles, Editor, Second Edition, Glaxo Inc., Research Triangle Park, NC. 1991.

Glaxo Pathway Evaluation Program for Pharmacy Professionals: Specialty Profiles/ Career Options, Editor, First Edition, Glaxo Inc., Research Triangle Park, NC. 1990.

Quick Order Form

Internet orders: www.thegoodpharmacist.com (best method)

Fax orders: (727)786-3424 (next best method)

Postal orders: 2147 Warwick Drive, Oldsmar, FL 34677 (slowest method)

Email orders with this form as an attachment to: wnkelly@earthlink.net
(ok method)

No. of Copies @ $16.95 ($17.95 Canada) + postage & handling $3.25/
copy ($5.00 Canada)

PLEASE PRINT OR TYPE

Name: _____

Address (PO Box address is not acceptable) _____

City: _____ State/Province: _____

Country: _____ Zip/Postal Code: _____

Phone: _____

Attention: _____

Email: _____

Number of copies ordered: _____ PO # (if applicable): _____

Total price for books: $ _____ (bulk pricing is available on 20 or
more copies)

Total price for shipping and handling: $ _____

Total Cost: $ _____

Method of Payment (check one):

Check _____ Money Order _____ American Express _____

VISA _____ Master Card _____ Discover _____

Pay Pal _____

Card or Account Number: _____

CCV Code: _____

MX CCV Code: ____ ____ ____ ____

Expiration Date: ____ ____ ____

Name on Card: _____

Satisfaction Guaranteed